Proof of Concept

25 Best Cancer Cases
Presented to the
National Cancer Institute

by

Nicholas J. Gonzalez, M.D.

Notice

This book is intended for general informational purposes only, not as a medical manual. The materials presented in no way are meant to be a substitute for professional medical care or attention by a qualified practitioner, nor should they be construed as such. Always check with your doctor if you have any questions or concerns about your condition or before starting or modifying a program of treatment. New Spring Press LLC and the author(s) are not responsible or liable, directly or indirectly, for any form of damages whatsoever resulting from the use (or misuse) of information contained in or implied by this book.

Book design by Six Penny Graphics

Cover design by Six Penny Graphics

Dedication

This book is being published four years after Dr. Nicholas Gonzalez's passing on July 21st 2015 so we don't have the benefit of his decision as to whom he would dedicate this book. However, there is only one person who stood by Nick during the first years of his private medical practice and helped him prepare this career-changing presentation in 1993 to the National Cancer Institute. That same person helped Nick with the resulting clinical trial and worked in the office trenches with him for more than 25 years. Nick was very grateful for this support.

I dedicate *Proof of Concept* to Dr. Linda Isaacs for her devoted service to Nick and their patients.

Mary Beth Gonzalez

Contents

Foreword

By Linda L. Isaacs, M.D.

This monograph provides an additional piece of documentation of the accomplishments of a remarkable man, my long-time colleague and friend, the late Dr. Nicholas Gonzalez. Nick had been successful in the world of journalism before he decided, in his late 20s, to become a physician. While in medical school, he encountered the work of Dr. William Donald Kelley, an orthodontist who had developed a nutritional method for the treatment of cancer and other illnesses. Nick dedicated his life to preserving this treatment method and to trying to get it properly scientifically evaluated.

Nick's findings among Dr. Kelley's patient records would eventually be published, 25 years later, as the book One Man Alone.[1] But at the time Nick finished his investigation of Dr. Kelley's records in 1986, no journal editor or book publisher was willing to accept that the case reports were real, or to take the risk of antagonizing others in the medical world. I was already working with Nick at that time; I remember the numerous submissions of case reports and manuscripts, which we painstakingly printed, feeding one sheet at a time to a noisy daisy-wheel printer. I remember disappointment building as the rejections came. Finally, Dr. Kelley began to mistrust us, and it became clear that Nick and I could no longer work with him. Since Dr. Kelley was no longer seeing patients, Nick decided that he should try to recreate the protocol, in the hope of collecting new patient success stories to further document that the treatment could work, and that someone other than Dr. Kelley could implement it.

In the fall of 1987, Nick began seeing patients in New York City, in the office of a physician friend. Even though I had finished medical school and internship and could get a medical license, there was nowhere for me to see patients, so I helped out administratively until I resumed my internal medicine residency in June 1989. Those were difficult times; our resources were limited, but there was much to be done. Nick wrote instructions for diets and detoxification protocols, decided what supplements to use, and figured out how to get them distributed. He had to get the word out that he was seeing patients, using contacts such as Dr. Robert Atkins, whom Nick had once interviewed for a magazine article when he was a journalist. Most challenging of all was patient care. We had to learn the hard way the limitations of the treatment method and of our own stamina. In the early days, Nick was making house calls on patients who in retrospect were simply too ill to benefit. Both Nick and I were tempted on many occasions to quit, but invariably, when we were despondent over one poor outcome, shortly afterwards we would get good news about another patient who was improving.

In 1991, I finished my internal medicine residency and passed my boards. I rejoined Nick, but there was still no room for me to see patients in the office he rented. While Nick saw patients,

I reviewed his charts, looking for remarkable outcomes and incomplete records, sending out requests for records from other treating physicians, radiology facilities, and hospitals. All this proved invaluable when Nick was invited to present a Best Case Series in 1993 at the National Cancer Institute.

For his presentation, Nick was determined that every detail would be in place. We felt a single bit of missing data could provide an excuse for someone to criticize his selected cases. It became my mission to track down actual X-ray and CT films, to get pathology slides, and to be sure every relevant document was included. Meanwhile, Nick continued to work long hours seeing patients and returning phone calls, while writing the monograph that is being published here. We had it printed and bound, and distributed it to the attendees at his presentation, with medical records included so that no one could question the patients' diagnoses. In this era, before the draconian HIPAA requirements came into play, we were able to leave patient names and identifying information intact for the government scientists to see.

In his introduction to this monograph, Nick discussed supporting evidence for the treatment, including the work of Dr. John Beard, who first suggested that pancreatic enzymes could be used to treat cancer.[2] Beard's thesis centered on the similarity in appearance and behavior of cancer cells to the trophoblast, the earliest stage of the mammalian placenta. Beard had observed that the trophoblast moderated its aggressive, invasive nature around the time the fetus began making pancreatic enzymes. He speculated that pancreatic enzymes could also moderate the behavior of cancer, which he felt arose from "aberrant" trophoblast cells that were retained in adult tissues as a reservoir for repair—similar to the function of what are now called stem cells. At the time of Nick's NCI presentation in 1993, little of this was corroborated in the scientific literature, but now the similarity of the trophoblast to cancer is widely recognized.[3,4] On a molecular level, receptors for proteolytic pancreatic enzymes have been found on both trophoblast and cancer cells.[5,6] Even without the knowledge of Beard's unifying theory about pancreatic enzymes, research is proceeding that may eventually bring modern science to the same conclusions Beard made more than a century ago.

Nick also included references on the therapeutic use of enemas in his presentation; a recent article documents the usefulness of coffee enemas in stimulating bile flow, corroborating what Dr. Kelley and others had claimed as the mechanism of action of this detoxification technique.[7]

While Nick went to make his presentation in Bethesda, MD, I stayed in New York to manage patient calls. I still remember watching him leave, trundling a heavy collection of radiology films on a luggage cart, filled with hope and optimism. Looking back 25 years later, I am amazed that Nick was able to put together this case series after only six years in practice. We have never seen high volumes of patients; it takes time to collect the information needed to design protocols for our patients, time to explain it, and time to return the phone calls to answer patients' questions. And the patients in this volume were not the only patients in the practice doing well. There were some who simply were not far enough out from diagnosis in 1993 to be reportable cases.

The scientists in attendance at Nick's presentation suggested a pilot study looking at pancreatic cancer, though no funding was provided to facilitate it. We began that work in 1994; by that time, we had moved into a larger office where I too could see patients. What happened next has been documented elsewhere; the results of the pilot study were published in 1999,[8] followed by the mismanaged clinical trial that concluded in 2005, a bitter disappointment to both of us.[9,10] But throughout our time in practice, even as our formal research efforts bogged down in a miasma of mismanagement and indifference from the academic world, we continued to have patients doing well. We published a collection of case reports in 2007,[11] and Nick was working on a large collection of them at the time of his death, subsequently published as Conquering Cancer: Volumes One and Two.[12,13] Some of the patient stories described in this monograph are continued in those books. Some of the patients are still alive.

It is still hard to believe, four years later, that Nick is no longer here. But I continue seeing patients, as I know he would want, and I continue to see patients do well. I plan, in due time, to continue to publish case reports, in the hope that someday the work that Dr. Kelley, Nick and I did will get the vindication Nick never got during his life. And I find encouragement to continue from the passionate gratitude of the patients, both his and mine, whose lives have been transformed by the methods Nick fought so hard to preserve.

1. Gonzalez NJ. *One Man Alone; An Investigation of Nutrition, Cancer, and William Donald Kelley.* New York, NY: New Spring Press; 2010.
2. Beard J. *The Enzyme Treatment of Cancer and Its Scientific Basis.* London: Chatto and Windus; 1911.
3. Murray MJ, Lessey BA. Embryo implantation and tumor metastasis: common pathways of invasion and angio-genesis. *Semin Reprod Endocrinol.* 1999;17(3):275–290.
4. Gonzalez NJ, Isaacs LL. *The Trophoblast and the Origins of Cancer: One solution to the medical enigma of our time.* New York, NY: New Spring Press; 2009.
5. Bar-Shavit R, Maoz M, Kancharla A, et al. Protease-activated receptors (PARs) in cancer: Novel biased signaling and targets for therapy. *Methods Cell Biol.* 2016;132:341–358.
6. Even-Ram SC, Grisaru-Granovsky S, Pruss D, et al. The pattern of expression of protease-activated receptors (PARs) during early trophoblast development. *J Pathol.* 2003;200(1):47–52.
7. Kim ES, Chun HJ, Keum B, et al. Coffee enema for preparation for small bowel video capsule endoscopy: a pilot study. *Clinical nutrition research.* 2014;3(2):134–141.
8. Gonzalez NJ, Isaacs LL. Evaluation of pancreatic proteolytic enzyme treatment of adenocarcinoma of the pancre-as, with nutrition and detoxification support. *Nutr Cancer.* 1999;33(2):117–124.
9. Isaacs LL. Research Battles: Survival Tips From a Veteran. *Integr Med (Encinitas).* 2015;14(5):30–32.
10. Gonzalez NJ. *What Went Wrong: The Truth Behind the Clinical Trial of the Enzyme Treatment of Cancer.* New York, NY: New Spring Press; 2012.
11. Gonzalez NJ, Isaacs LL. The Gonzalez therapy and cancer: a collection of case reports. *Altern Ther Health Med.* 2007;13(1):46–55.
12. Gonzalez NJ. *Conquering Cancer: Volume One.* New York, NY: New Spring Press; 2016.
13. Gonzalez NJ. *Conquering Cancer: Volume Two.* New York, NY: New Spring Press; 2017.

Preface

By Faiz Khan, M.D.

In reading about and speaking with people who knew Dr. Nicholas Gonzalez well—I find myself taken on a tour of what it means to be a dedicated physician scientist. This was brilliantly exemplified through his remarkable work.

There is a saying that: *it is hard to see the fallacy in an enterprise when your paycheck depends on NOT seeing it.* And for those who do see it, *it is just as hard to walk away from a false enterprise when your paycheck depends on you NOT walking away.*

Now, dare I say that conventional approaches to cancer treatment are categorically false? No—of course not. Very few things are categorically false. Dr. Gonzalez himself yielded that in a minority of cancers—there was a role from chemotherapy and other conventional modalities. This was a tiny minority. For the most part—conventional treatments for cancer have been a tremendous disappointment compared to the approaches Gonzalez not only adopted from great minds before him, but further advanced. His journey revealed important considerations about the current landscape of modern medical practice.

In looking at his professional life's encounters—we can see a difference between what I would call the "health care industry" or conventional medical industry versus those remnant physicians who truly represent what can be called a dedicated medical profession. On what grounds does this dichotomy exist? Well, unbeknownst to many physicians and of course the lay public, conventional medical approaches are not based strictly on scientific merit, nor on putting the patients consideration first.[1] Two main factors lie behind this problematic dynamic. One has to do with a defect in conventional medical education—and the other factor which partially contributes to this defect, , is the cartel dynamic of the medical industry. Both have a common denominator. This denominator is financial hegemony.

The cartel consists of elements within a network of third party payors, the medical service sector, and the regulative enitities (professional boards and governmental agencies). The third party payors (who call themselves insurance or benefits programs) are those who pre- appropriate the dollars from you and me that are supposed to pay for medical expenses.[2] The service side is composed of facilities, technologies, pharmaceuticals, and of course the physicians and their supporting personnel—all of whom are directed to practice in a particular manner—if they are to be reimbursed for their efforts. And one more component is the regulatory arm (government and medical boards)—which ultimately deem what is and is not acceptable medical practice.

---

1   The latter may seem like an alarming statement, but unfortunately this is how the conventional medical industry has evolved. The lack of patient centeredness can be readily felt or seen in many realms of health care 'delivery'— ranging from the mazes of self-serving bureaucracies patients need to navigate to even access proper medical care, to the way new treatments are either rushed onto 'market' or the opposite—restricted from 'the market.'
2   These are the 'premiums' mandated to be taken from your earnings every month.

When we examine 'the particular manner' in which physicians are indoctrinated or even coerced to practice, as mentioned above—it is not based strictly on scientific merit. The 'education' medical students and training physicians receive is heavily influenced by—and hence feeds, the industry. Any modalities discovered (disruptive innovation)which effectively combat disease (through treatment or real cure) in a manner far superior to what the industry, or what is at times labeled as 'standard of care' offers is dismissed through a variety of means.

So the two main factors mentioned above which sustain a medical industry that finds itself at cross purposes with a dedicated medical profession are (1) the very curricula/indoctrination program that is used to educate physicians and (2) the cartel which dominates medical services. The most immediate cartel factor for the public is the third party payors who take their cue from the industry; these payors who have taken our premium dollars have the power to allocate those dollars to only certain services and treatment modalities—despite their lack of efficacy or even scientific merit when scrutinized through an authentic scientific analysis, And despite the availability of clearly efficacious treatments for chonic diseases for which payment should be provided if policies were based on sanity, commitment to stated mission, and patient centeredness.

Now the 'regulation' of the conventional medical curricula that teaches the 'menu' of services deemed to be worthy to offer by the conventional medical industry—began to take form in the early 20th century with the Flexner report; enough has been written about the dynamics behind this report and the reader is welcome to explore this. Composed by a man named Abraham Flexner, the result of this report was a limiting of what federal and state legislative bodies would accept as proper practice under a medical license. Most folks do not know that Flexner was not doctor. He was a school teacher and education theorist. The report was commissioned by financiers and industrialists (Carnegie, Rockefeller, Morgan—to name a few. These folks were heavily invested in the menu that they thought should dominate the industry). Diagnostic and treatment modalities that were outside 'the menu, ' yet still had an effective track record for centuries and even millennia were considered 'outside of sound medical practice'—many such practitioners and training institutions were shut down forcibly.

Looking at the landscape from a strictly scientific perspective: What we have today in conventional medical education is an indoctrination process that suffers from two issues; the first is paradigmatic, and the second is epistemic.

Paradigmatically speaking—conventional medical education is incomplete:[3] On the level of physiology, pathophysiology and treatment options—many elements are missing or not covered in a thorough manner. For example—a proper study of nutrition and nutrient priming, the prevalence of environmental toxins (metals, metalloids, xenobiotics, organic pollutants, endocrine disruptors), nutrient depletion states, detox modalities for chronic illnesses, biophysics/electromagnetic diagnostics and treatments, novel and natural anti-septics and immune modulators, lymphatic and chiropractic techniques, gut rehabilitation, autonomic nervous system balancing using the medicinal properties of herbs, whole foods and their pure extracts , more subtle cybernetic approaches such as homeopathy, and much more. Even president Richard Nixon could not help but marvel at the bio-electromagnetic modality known as acupuncture and explicitly encouraged its acceptance into formal medical training. It is no wonder that many of the

---

3   This is slowly changing as conventional medical schools are including complementary/alternative medicine modules in their training. The recent 'functional medicine' movement is a reaction to the recognized inadequacies in conventional medical education. However compared to the rigors of what proper science and dedication to the task of healing would dictate—there is still an unfortunate large gap.

greatest integrative physicians who have paved the way for fields such as homeopathy, naturopathy, bioenergetics, regenerative medicine—did so after the inadequacies they faced through their MD training when confronting chronic diseases in the real world. In addition—their dilemma led to great enhancements in the adoption of novel therapies that were not necessarily a product of the pharmaceutical industry. The fascinating and effective use of ozone and silver is one such example. In all fairness—although conventional medicine is pharmaceutical and tech/operative intervention dominant, and tends to be more reductionist in its approach to analyzing a disease state; despite this—in all cases I recall during my conventional medical education—mention was always made of the need for 'supportive care' which was necessary to accompany any conventional intervention. This to me is an allusion to the holistic side of treatment strategies and using some of the above-mentioned factors to enhance the body's endogenous regenerative capacity. The phrase *supportive care* is almost never taken nor practiced in this manner however.

It should also be mentioned that there are hosts of well-meaning but unqualified or even frank charlatans who take advantage of the obvious limits of conventional medicine. They attain some sort of certification, 'raise the flag', publicize, and claim to implement many of the above mentioned non-conventional modalities. They do so in an incompetent fashion. The result of their attempts to offer patients an 'alternative' to what they always preach is a monolithically bad conventional medical approach is either no effect, or even dangerous outcome (many such patients have ended up in my ER)—and hence such modalities receive a poor reputation; the conventional industry wastes no time in celebrating such failures. This is why a seeker should find a true integrative physician or team of such—because no one paradigm or approach has a monopoly on healing everything which may ail the human body. The proper balance between reductionist and holistic conceptualizations are necessary to both understand and treat disease states—instead of a categorical blindness to either.

In addition to the limitations in actual modalities of treatment—mention must be made with regard to the very paradigms that are used to *conceptualize* the well state and disease state. A severe myopia exists in the conventional medical world with regard to not fully understanding (or perhaps refusing to acknowledge) the cybernetic multidimensionality of of human homeostasis, pathophysiology, and the human regenerative capacity. This term cybernetic is extremely apt and connotes 'communication, information, and control systems.' From this perspective—human homeostasis is a breathtaking cybernetic system. We find dizzying exchanges of information— command, control, feedback, execution, response, monitoring—and more; all happening more than trillions of times per second ranging at levels from the photonic, electronic, microscopic to macro and gross means.; however reducing such to thermodynamic ligand receptor models, diffusion gradients, bumping of molecules, and even ionic transfers—in light of empirical observations is at best a modern superstition. Sure these elements do indeed exist AND can be harnessed for diagnostic and therapeutic purposes—but if it is taught that the same mechanisms that can make a frog's leg twitch in a petri dish filled with salt solution, is the same which allows something even so routine as the visual faculty's ability to maintain a dynamic visual field array, (let alone the billions of homeostatic interactions, or even consciousness) then I am afraid an intellectual castration of a horrible sort is going on.[4]

The incomplete understanding of physiology and pathophysiology errs in looking at signs and symptoms of a given problem from a narrow perspective, and thus remains blind to effecting real restorative treatment. One of the unfortunate consequences of this incomplete perspective is

---

4   See chapters 4 and 5 of Science and Myth by Dr. Wolfgang Smith PhD, Angelico Press/Sophia Perennis ,2010.

seeking an 'antidote' model for a given disease state. Conventional medicine is dominated by a quest to find a synthetic chemical to put in the body that will 'neutralize' the problem.[5] It allows for invasive procedures to 'remove the problem.' Or—it does allow for the use of electromagnetic energy to destroy the problem (or in the case of electroconvulsive therapy or cardioversion … re-calibrate the problematic system). Now there are clearly times where this is appropriate—but in most chronic disorders for most of their natural arcs of time—it is NOT effective.[6] Some of these may palliate symptoms, but other symptoms come to the forefront, and there are of course subversive effects of these interventions. Meanwhile the underlying disease state advances. A real regenerative process is not fostered to heal or cure.

Another important element to understand with respect to the paradigmatic climate in conventional medicine is what I would call the 'chasing of phantasms' when it comes to seeking more and more chemicals to throw at various phase reactants in disease states—be they to the latest genetic codon expression, or interleukin, cytokine, fancy receptor, protein marker, chemokine, ultrakines… etc.[7] To do this rests on two very flimsy suppositions—and the track record of using this approach demonstrates practically no clinically meaningful outcomes . . Reliable good clinical outcomes are the gold standard against which anything must be evaluated. This is a most neglected concept and its neglect will be elaborated further in discussion.

The first supposition leading to the 'chasing of phantasms' states that we have elucidated enough of the domain in a particular disease state, such that: given a known pathophysiologic cascade of phase reactants, we may manipulate one or more reactants to eliminate the problem and perhaps the disease state. To assume the full landscape is what you see through a peep-hole symbolizes this problem nicely. The supposition of course is continuously found to be false—and the term "irreducible complexity" has arisen precisely because we bump into the fact that we keep learning more and more about how less and less of a complete picture we have within a given domain of pursuit (be it molecular genetics, or physical chemistry), and we note how less and less we are able to neatly 'concretize' human biology when it comes to probing disease states exclusively on the level of physical chemistry, biochemistry, molecular biology and its related sub-disciplines. I am reminded of the term 'physics envy.' This describes the mental deficiency that fails to recognize the limitation that arises from thinking about chronic diseases states in too schematic or compartmentalized a fashion—as one would when approaching physics (on a macro level such as kinematics or electromagnetic dynamics) or as one would when approaching chemistry or organic chemistry. To be sure these are important foundations that have an absolute heuristic value—but to assume that on this level of a given pathophysiology—one could exhaustively map the conditions is bordering on the absurd. And in addition—to think pathophysiology exists exclusively on such a level is even more absurd.[8]

I recall being a panelist during a debate about emerging stem cell technologies from an ethical point of view. Of course it was an ideologically charged issue—and if folks understood the actual

---

5   This is how the public sees it and it is a pharmaceutical bias which many physicians hold. It is based on the antibiotic model; antibiotics are extremely effective and lifesaving when they are used appropriately; they neutralize the pathos; however other pharmaceuticals are NOT potions which resolve or neutralize causes—except in a minority of situations. Constantly however—the public looks for an antidote to their given symptom complex/disease.

6   I have often explained to patients—unless you really need (emphasis on 'really need') an ER, OR, or ICU, or palliation of pain—there is very little that conventional medicine can offer to improve your condition.

7   Simply a logical extension of the isolated reductionist myopia

8   And this physics envy becomes even more comedic when it is seen in fields such as psychology, sociology, economics, politics—all of which hastily attach the term 'science' onto their respective fields of study.

science it would have been less so—since real progress has been made through adult stem cells (versus the controversial embryonic) and the exosome features in their matrices/supernatants. But during one segment a particular bench researcher put up a nice dizzying schematic diagram of how this magic bullet or few bullets would work,…with the metabolic pathways neatly lableled with catchy designs—whizzing around and receptors waking up and launching their signals… how we could target all of those to synthesize more neurotranmitters (assuming cognition could be boiled down to 'not enough neurotransmitters' or even neurotranmitters period) …etc. in reversing dementia. After all of the oohs and aahs—I had to play the intelligent contrarian and share the fact that the schematic itself was more a product of fantasy than any real assessment. Such oversimplified reductionist views are not uncommon in approaching therapeutics for chronic disease. My position should NOT be misunderstood. There is great value in elucidating biochemical and histologic pathways—but my point can be illustrated in the following metaphor: Given that we have limited resources—Let us assume that we have to figure out a way to cross an ocean more efficiently than by boat; we have two plausible scenarios; Dr. A is working on a giant power sling-shot to propel a pod of passengers. His power point images with dizzying and impressive schematics show that material science supports the idea that with the right combination of tensile strength and elasticity ratios, and given the right launch angle and aerodynamic modeling of the pod—the pod can get across. Dr. B posits that combustion seen in the natural world can be induced and harnessed to power a craft—and the power generated can get the craft across. Both put up their impressive schematic diagrams that demonstrate plausibility.

Now after how many trials of each are we going to divert full resources to Dr. B?

The second supposition that perpetuates the 'chasing of phantasms' is related to this first. We suppose that our proposed solution contains within it the sufficient degree of complexity to match that of the stage/level in which we choose to engage the problematic condition. More specifically: Given that we limit ourselves to a particular domain of a pathophysiologic problem, [9] we suppose that we are able to match the complexity in the solution against the existing degree of complexity on that particular domain of the pathophysiologic process. The flaw in this second assumption requires further explanation that will now proceed.

One of the axioms in approaching a given problem within a cybernetic system is the following: a solution for a problem at a given stage requires the same amount of informational complexity (bits of solution or 'neutralizing' or 'control' information) as are contained at the given stage or level of the problem. This is common sense. If all five elements that make up a given problem need to be neutralized for the problem to disappear—my solution better have the 'complexity' which holds the five neutralizing capacities. If 5 bowling pins need to be knocked down—my solution better contain the complexity which would enable such to happen, either by launching 5 different projectiles with respective trajectories, or by rolling a large ball with sufficiently programmed motion through use of my forearm, wrist musculature. So if there are two dozen *dynamic* variables (far more challenging than dealing with static elements (bowling pins) as mentioned in the prior sentence)—variables which adapt, re-route, evade, and counter-measure in order to maintain a pathologic homeostasis—and these are perpetuating a problem at the level which we choose to engage the condition—, and we pride ourselves in throwing a chemical dart or two at that level— what are we to expect of this logic? Again—my words should not be misunderstood. We can hope to get lucky and measure the clinical outcomes of such an attempt. But are we surprised when

---

9   level and stage

these outcomes reveal no meaningful improvements, except by torturing statistical methods (as we shall mention further on) What if there are more than the two dozen, which we have erroneously assumed to be the complete view? Well then the situation is even direr.[10]

In the end—I suggest the following , and as such, I simply affirm a perennial wisdom found in the field of medicine: Given the raw materials and energetic state a system needs, a biological system which is characterized by a profound cybernetic aimed at homeostasis will adapt in the wisest way possible for a given set of stressors, or… more hopefully—regenerate as much as possible .. In case of humans—a biological system includes molecular, electromagnetic, and psychologic.[11] The key to real regenerative medical therapeutics is to *feed the regenerative capacity*. This stands in contradistinction to trying to micromanage its multileveled complexity, or even stand in, or substitute for it.

So one may ask—if the modern approach violates so many paradigmatic axioms—how does the industry perpetuate itself? In a few words: Propaganda plus frank restrictive imposition from the above mentioned cartel behavior of the medical industry.

I use the term propaganda in its purest sense. Of course two levels of propaganda exist: one targets those minds that demonstrate an aptitude superior enough to gain entry into conventional medical education. The other target is of course the laity—which now gets it's dose of propaganda thanks to the unfortunate legislation that has allowed the pharmaceutical industry to directly access the lay media.

---

10 I am reminded of an illustrative example of this misguidance, namely the continual attempts to pretend that such a magic bullet exists when approaching the condition known as severe sepsis or septic shock. Mainstays of therapy included supportive measures (nutrient priming and hemodynamic support) plus interventions which target the simpler levels of pathophysiology (from a cybernetic perspective): namely etiology source control via excision or antibiotics. Nevertheless, over 25 years plus of practice I witnessed the incessant roll-outs of the 'chemical du jour ' which promised to be the next amazing adjunct—and predictably they have thus far been failures. They do get their false moment in the sun based on some study which tortures the outcomes data statistically to barely move the odds ratio in favor of survival—and hence attributes this to the magic bullet intervention. The same 'play' happens in conventional oncology I am afraid. So any intervention which has made a significant impact on survival in the sepsis model has attacked the problem at a proximal point where the cybernetic simplicity allows neutralization of the pathos and cure. It should be noted that the only recent modality which has demonstrated a large treatment effect and outcome changes has been Vitamin C in super therapeutic doses. For a variety of reasons this has not been embraced. However it's efficacy makes sense in light of what has been discussed about cybernetics—it feeds the endogenous reactive, adaptive and subsequent regenerative capacity of human physiology. It does not seek to micromanage it or substitute for it. For in this latter approach arises a complexity which outdoes any current attempt to comprehensively master it—to the extent where we can 'stand in ' for it. This further brings to mind what critical care experts have known and what a sage intensivist mentor taught me long ago; a teaching that corresponds to how Dr. Gonzalez approached his treatment of advanced cancer. This teaching dictated: don't mess with the bodies reactive, adaptive, and regenerative 'moves.' Simply support them. He said this in two contexts: one—"always use the gut for nutrition whenever possible"—because we can never micromanage nutrient delivery into the system like the gut can. And the second—'don't mess with the brainstem.' This means that to assume you know where a blood pressure should be, or a respiratory rate should be, or a heart rate should be, or even a temperature should be—better than a patients intact brainstem—is the height of stupidity. Yet here we stand—with a multibillion dollar industry convincing the medical community and lay public to chase BP numbers which they have defined as 'optimal' (the standards which just happen to keep on changing to diagnose more and more with the specter of hypertension.) Here we stand—stamping out fevers left and right to psychologically assuage ourselves and uneducated moms—because somehow the irrational meme that *to bring down fever must be good* still has a grip on the modern psyche.

11 I use the term psychologic in the original sense of the term 'psyche'—meaning that particular faculty of the human being which equates for 'soul' (greek: psyche, latin: animus', hebrew/arabic: nefs; vedic: atman). This latter term has become so problematic with the advent of the intellectual castration and reflexive hostility arisen from the various flavors of modernist ideologies—that the term psyche has lost it's precision and even validity in terms of effectuating primary etiologic pathos on a physiologic level.

So the former level of propaganda, which validates flawed or ineffective therapeutic approaches to chronic disease—this level comes in the guise of 'science.' And the young minds go through the curriculum trusting that what they receive intellectually is 'settled science,'—or rather—the 'best possible evidence.' Now there stands a monumental level of analysis, documentation, and proof that such is not the case. The epistemic basis used to validate conventional approaches to chronic disease suffers from hosts of fallacies. We already discussed questionable paradigmatic assumptions. It would be beyond the scope of this essay to fully elucidate the holes in the epistemic and specific research methodologies that are used to justify the various dogmas AND to disqualify valid conclusions—but they range from: outright fraud and malfeasance, false assumptions between virtual/ vitro modeling and in vivo conditions, various levels of prevalent bias (both ignorant or complicit), internal and external invalidities of study designs, ecologic and atomistic fallacies embedded within conclusions, neglect of multidimensional causal logic— and my favorite: the outright torture or wrongful application of aggregate statistical inferential methods in analyzing outcomes. This is well known and called 'pushing and pulling' the statistical methods with the intention of demonstrating an outcome difference between a trial group and control group—and then attributing that outcome to the intervention. Pertaining to this latter— one expert rightly said that there is a pandemic of ignorance amongst medical professionals when it comes to making conclusions about etiologics and in evaluating therapeutic approaches. How does such ignorance attain prevalence? Most physicians are illiterate when it comes to methods of statistical validation—and the ones that propagate the pseudo-dogmas that arise from such methods are not sufficiently literate enough with regard to the logical limits of aggregate statistical inference (or are dis-incentivized to pursue dubious conclusions with proper rigor). Just where a sound conclusion stops and delusional speculative dogma begins remains ambiguous in the minds of the alleged experts. Again—the severely impaired teach the completely impaired. [12] The result is a delusional over certainty about what is valid AND delusional over certainty about what should be disqualified. If any a reader feels that what I am conveying sounds too fantastic (and tragic) to accept—they are free to once again re-visit my background credentials at the introduction of this essay, and furthermore investigate the matter themselves in take into considerations the ensuing words:

In the words of Dr. Marcia Angell—Faculty MD at Harvard, "It is simply no longer possible to believe much of the clinical research that is published, or to rely on the judgment of trusted physicians or authoritative medical guidelines. I take no pleasure in this conclusion, which I reached slowly and reluctantly over my two decades as an editor of The New England Journal of Medicine." The New England Journal of Medicine is considered the most prestigious medical journal in the nation. Dr. Angell was Time Magazine's top 25 influential Americans in 1997 and Master of the American College of Physicians. She is also author of the book: *The Truth About the Drug Companies: How They Deceive Us and What to Do About It* (Random House 2005).

Furthermore, in *Why Most Published Research Findings Are False*, Dr. John Ioannidis states *"Evidence-based medicine has been hijacked:"* John P. A. Ioannidis MD is a Stanford Research Expert. He estimates 90% of studies are flawed enough to call conclusions doubtful.

---

12 William Matthew ("Matt") Briggs, Ph.D.: Statistical Follies and Epidemiology. https://www.youtube.com/ watch?v=C42AwvaZ-04

The Crisis Of Evidence, Or, Why Probability & Statistics Cannot Discover Cause https://www.youtube.com/ watch?v=rbf_TXqEY-Y

Uncertainty: The Soul of Modeling, Probability & Statistics—Springer Press, 2016

Now that we covered propaganda—we make brief reference to the other dynamic which keeps the impairment functioning—the medical industry cartel. Brief mention was made of this dynamic at the outset—and many authors and journalists have elucidated the various types of harms and restrictions that this structure imposes on both physicians and the public at large. Here we will only make mention of the natural outcome of such which pertains to perpetuating the limitations of therapeutic choices for the public. A cartel seeks to 'corner' a service market—and hence does its best to make sure anything outside "it's menu" is unavailable. This state of affairs really is no surprise to those who have lived in this world long enough. It must be said at the outset that most involved in the cartel structure of the medical industry are generally well meaning and sincere individuals. It has however, now grown to collusion between financial entities, industry providers (tech/big pharma, medical institutions and governing bodies), and 3ʳᵈ party payors (benefits programs/insurance companies). The results is that physicians are indoctrinated into a practice which creates demand for the *industry menu*—and physicians are more and more serving as employees of this industry, due to the pressures directly and indirectly linked from the industry against independent practice AND thinking. The industry menu dominates the modern conventional medical education curricula, so generations of medical students know little else BUT to implement demand for the industry menu. Where this truly benefits patients this is fine but where this works to restrict physicians from acquiring intellectual and technical skills that would provide effective therapies for the public—this is damaging. As far as quality goes—conventional industry medicine works best in the emergency rooms, operating rooms, and intensive care units. But for disease states in their chronic or sub-acute form—unfortunately not only does the cartel have very little to offer—it works to suppress effective alternatives on one hand and exaggerate it's claims in the setting of chronic disease on the other.

Within the conventional cancer sector we observe the same dynamics at work. *Exaggerate the merits of your own menu, and discredit any other menu.* This is done on the level of the paradigmatic and epistemics by either the abovementioned pseudo research, or pseudo-interpretations using sleights of hand—that serve to validate or invalidate in the desired direction.

"My overall assessment is that the national cancer program must be judged a qualified failure" Dr. John Bailer, who spent 20 years on the staff of the U.S. National Cancer Institute and was editor of its journal.

Dr. Bailer also says: "The five year survival statistics of the American Cancer Society are very misleading. They now count things that are not cancer, and, because we are able to diagnose at an earlier stage of the disease, patients falsely appear to live longer. Our whole cancer research in the past 20 years has been a total failure. More people over 30 are dying from cancer than ever before... More women with mild or benign diseases are being included in statistics and reported as being 'cured'. *When government officials point to survival figures and say they are winning the war against cancer they are using those survival rates improperly."* (3) Dr. Bailer, speaking at the Annual Meeting of the American Association for the Advancement of Science in May 1985.

"Everyone should know that most cancer research is largely a fraud and that the major cancer research organizations are derelict in their duties to the people who support them." Linus Pauling PhD (Two-time Nobel Prize winner).

"There is not one, but many cures for cancer available. But they are all being systematically suppressed by the ACS (American Cancer Society), the NCI (National Cancer Institute) and the major oncology centers. They have too much of an interest in the status quo."—Dr. Robert Atkins, M.D.

There are of course other ways to eliminate an alternative menu from the minds of physicians and the lay. Unfortunately—the incidence of cancer overall and in the young is rising at an alarming rate. In the 1970's overall incidence was roughly 1 in 10; currently it's closer to 1 in 3. This is despite the billions spent. The analysis of survival time from onset of diagnoses is riddled with ambiguities, claims and counter claims. Moreover, if accurate statistics were obtainable—there are severe problems in making comparisons year to year due to the massive heterogeneity amongst cases. Dr. Gonzalez nicely discusses the difficulty in using population/aggregate epidemiology and statistics in deriving valid conclusions. This is referred to in a later section. And once more in terms of 'limiting the menu,' ultimately from a practical and material level—recall that the conventional industry can control the menu options by dictating what will and will NOT be paid for.

So enter Dr. Nicholas Gonzalez into this landscape. He faced all of the above mentioned hurdles on the landscape of the conventional medical approaches and industry. Like other superb medical doctors before him—he rejected the fallacies and defective paradigms and sought science and real clinical outcomes based approaches to guide his therapies. This has been the case for many physicians who, when confronted with the ineffectiveness of the menu offered by the conventional medical industry when it comes to chronic disease states—sought to find other more effective menus. This has always been a sign of serious advances in the medical world—replicable, reliable clinical outcomes that do not require mega trials, meta analyses, tortured statistics, misapplications of p values, overlooked ecological fallacies, and thousands of patients in each arm in order to move the likelihood ratios a few percentage points in favor of the menu. Finding a difference in 'noise' between an alleged control arm and intervention arm, and declaring that it is authentic 'signal' (effect) of a given intervention is a slight of hand that Dr. Gonzalez's reports did not require. The documentation Dr. Gonzalez provided with this respect on well-documented advanced cancer cases was stunning.

Enough has been written elsewhere about his life and work—so I will mention salient features that bear upon how effective his work was in dealing with the problematic landscape that is conventional medical industry. To begin with—from the perspective of the conventional medical world with respect to cancer management—his credentials were unassailable. Studies at Brown and Columbia gained him entry into one of the top medical schools in the country—Cornell University Medical School. Through his medical education and post graduate training in internal medicine and immunology, he was mentored by the most published author in the history of medicine—Dr. Robert Good MD—considered the 'father of immunology' and at that time director of the world famous Memorial Sloan Kettering cancer institute. So it can be stated with complete assurance that Dr. Gonzalez received the most superior training possible for the treatment of cancers; so much so that he was on the track to set up bone-marrow transplant services. In the 80's and 90's this was a prestigious and lucrative career path and easily within his grasp. So with respect to the prior metaphor—he had mastered the 'best menu' conventional medicine had to offer for cancer. Displaying honesty and integrity—he chose to put it aside and implement another. I suspect much like the child with respect to the emperor's new clothes—he saw the conventional medical industry as naked with respect to claims made about treatment of cancer.

The methods Gonzalez adopted contained all of the hallmarks of sound medical therapeutic paradigms discussed above. He combined using an exogenous agent AND stimulating the endogenous regenerative capacity of the human body. He applied the work of his predecessors (John Beard PhD, William Kelley DDS) who had soundly validated their work both through the merits of scientific plausibility AND most important, reliable clinical outcomes.[13] In applying the protocols he found to produce the best clinical outcomes—he advanced them and improved them. Reading his patient case history accounts is to enjoy a refreshing episode of real medical science progression.

When I look at the concepts behind his methods I see that they paradigmatically display the wisdom of a proper therapeutic approach. The malignancy (the actual cells/tumor mass) is after all—a symptom. The problem is an *abnormal signal* in the microenvironment that induces the malignant change. Unless measures are taken to turn off the signal—efforts will be incomplete. The presence of that signal in a particular micro-environment can be expressed and monitored for progress in various terms which all have the same pathophysiologic implication: we can use pH terms, electromagnetic polarity terms, redox terms, microbiologic terms…they all indicate presence of a signal that induces a cell still sufficiently immature to take on malignant characteristics in obedience of such a signal. In recognizing this—Gonzalez knew that the conventional menu of either 'cut, burn, or poison' the clump or clumps was severely limited. It was dangerously incomplete or could even worsen the condition. [14]

So conceptually speaking the only way to turn off the signal is to get the physiology back to 'factory settings'—which not only means optimize—but the implication is that such a setting means absence of signal. Of course this concept is behind his formation of the individualized diet and individualized supplementation arm. As progress is made—the regenerative arm often includes addressing the need for a proper psychological or psycho-spiritual state. This latter has nothing to do with parochial or sectarian evangelization. It DOES have to do with the field of psycho-physiology and its relation to inducing disease states.

The exogenous agents he found to stimulate the neutralization of the cancer were pharmacologic doses of pancreatic enzymes. There are several competing hypotheses for the mechanisms of action. Whether the effects have to do with a signal which the enzymes emit which halts the infiltrative process, or direct proteolytic action of the enzymes on the tumor cells, or proteolytic neutralization of the evasive factors cancer cells use to hide from the hosts immune system (nagalase is hypothesized to be one such factor), or all of these, or none of these—the clinical results stand clear. Moreover Gonzalez expressly found evidence that the enzymes do pass through the gut intact—which would be necessary to occur if trans gut mucosal absorption of intact enzyme had something to do with the therapeutic physiology. However; from an epistemic point of view—reliable clinical outcomes are the gold standard for validating a therapeutic approach. Results trump any ambiguity in a mechanism of action hypothesis. Gonzalez's outcomes were unmatched.

And once again in accord with a paradigmatic wisdom—to support both the regenerative capacity and the fall out of the malignancy neutralization—The Gonzalez Protocol® called for enhanced detoxification methods. Gonzalez's mentor Dr. Kelley explained that during the protocol—not only are the trillions of trashcans or toilets of your body's cell going to flush… the filter that is your liver, kidney, gut, and skin are going to receive the wastes downstream. In this light—anyone with a sound understanding of pathophysiology would agree that optimizing

---

13 The case books are comprised of: *One Man Alone, Conquering Cancer: Volumes 1* and *2* and *Proof Of Concept* (New Spring Press)—where 175 plus advanced poor prognosis cancer cases are presented with documented reversal. The scientifically validated mechanisms of action are described in the book—*The Trophoblast and the Origins of Cancer, Nutrition and the Autonomic Nervous System* (both by Dr. Nicholas Gonzalez)—and John Beard's (PhD)'s *The Enzyme Treatment of Cancer* (foreword by Dr. Gonzalez.)

14 This latter point is fully acknowledged by the conventional oncology industry.

their excretory capacity is required. These methods included the coffee enema—which has an established efficacy even in the conventional medical literature.

The clinical outcomes Dr. Gonzalez obtained did not go unnoticed—and the 'conventional industry' acknowledged this. What followed illustrates the unfortunate combination of epistemic sleight of hand and cartel behavior reviewed above. In 1998, a prospective study comparing The Gonzalez Protocol® to chemotherapy was proposed and funded involving Columbia University and the National Cancer institute. By the end (2005)—it was riddled with so many fallacies that no meaningful conclusions could be made. This was not just Dr. Gonzalez's opinion— independent auditors of the study (including the NIH) shared this view. Moreover—there was clearly documented evidence of bias and sabotage against concluding positive outcomes with The Gonzalez Protocol. The details are available in several sources.[15]

There had been further proposals—and I feel Dr. Gonzalez matured to the point that he felt that all of the validation documentation was already out there and sufficient. Not only sufficient—but far superior to what the conventional industry offered to validate its 'menu.' And this we find is precisely in accordance with correctly understanding the epistemic basis of validation that we reviewed at the outset of this essay. The understanding which is rare in conventional medicine, and substituted by what can only be described as a 'cultish superstition' suffering not only from defects in methodology and execution of research, but in a delusional application of aggregate statistical inference in drawing conclusions. I suspect that Gonzalez already knew this, but saw in 1993 when he presented his 25 Best Cancer Cases to the NCI and again in 1998 when he cooperated with the conventional industry to conduct the NCI/NIH clinical trial so that he could demonstrate that even by their validation methods, there was merit in the protocols. With proper oversight I suspect that he would have succeeded, which is why it took gross mismanagement to thwart the correct conclusion.

In what I believe to be two of his most brilliant essays (*Some Thoughts on Scientific Bias*[16] and *Statistics: Why Meaningful Statistics Cannot Be Generated From a Private Practice*[17]), Dr. Gonzalez responds to a sincere repeat attempt to probe The Gonzalez Protocol via the conventional industry validation techniques. His response once again highlights the proper way of thinking about what constitutes evidence for merit in the medical sciences. Reliable, good, clinical outcomes of sufficient (not disguised) effect size are all Gonzalez needs to show…and he did so beyond doubt.

Faiz Khan, M.D. attained dual boarded status in Emergency and Internal Medicine through an accelerated combined residency at Long Island Jewish Medical Center /Albert Einstein College of Medicine in New York City. There he earned the resident leadership award and the Sir William Osler teaching award as assistant professor and associate residency director.

Dr. Khan then joined the faculty at Hershey Medical Center / Penn State College of Medicine as director of the medical observation unit and assistant residency director for emergency medicine.

He proceeded to serve as Vice-Chair of Emergency Medicine at Nassau University Medical Center, East Meadow–NY, where he was site residency director in emergency medicine, and served as hospital director of

15 Some Thoughts about Scientific Bias by Dr. Nicholas Gonzalez https://thegonzalezprotocol.com/scientific-bias/
16 Some Thoughts about Scientific Bias by Dr. Nicholas Gonzalez https://thegonzalezprotocol.com/scientific-bias/
17 Statistics: Why Meaningful Statistics Cannot Be Generated From a Private Practice), http://www.alternative-therapies.com/openaccess/ATHM_21_2_Gonzalez.pdf; http://www.alternative-therapies.com/at/web_pdfs/gonzalez1.pdf

medical ethics. He received the "physician of excellence" award for his teaching at the Nassau County Fire/Police Academy's Emergency Medical System program. Dr. Khan also served as Director and Chair of Emergency Medicine for the Kingston Hospital / Health Alliance of Hudson Valley, NY.

Dr. Khan went on as a founding partner of CityMD—New York City's largest urgent care practice. He currently practices and serves as executive VP focusing on physician development.

Dr. Khan is a fellow of the American College of Emergency Physicians and American Academy of Emergency Medicine. He is a member of the American College for the Advancement of Medicine, American Academy of Environmental Medicine, and American Association of Physicians and Surgeons.

Evaluating Anecdotes and Case Reports

Originally printed in *Alternative Therapies* Mar/Apr 2007, Vol. 13, No.2.

By Linda L. Isaacs, M.D.

Stories are more memorable than statistics. Newspaper or magazine articles about some new chemotherapy for cancer will typically include an interview with a patient doing well on it. Web sites of alternative practitioners and clinics sometimes feature stories by or about patients describing their successful treatment. These stories can be very persuasive to readers, but some scientists dismiss such stories scornfully as "anecdotal" and therefore meaningless.

Case reports, which have been published in the medical literature for decades, are also stories—they are descriptions of individual patients with unusual presentations or outcomes. What distinguishes an anecdote from a case report? As one author puts it, "The term 'anecdotal evidence' connotes secondhand or poorly documented fact and should not be confused with case studies of individual patients that involve careful observation and recording of detail".[1]

Anecdotes and case reports cannot be used to definitively prove a therapy is effective. But case reports cannot be dismissed entirely. As a recent article stated, "Case reports and series have a high sensitivity for detecting novelty and therefore remain one of the cornerstones of medical progress; they provide many new ideas in medicine."[2]

Case reports are a way to reveal the unknown or describe the previously unrecognized. They were critically important in the discovery of new diseases such as AIDS[3] or Lyme disease.[4]

Descriptions of sick birds and sick people helped scientists figure out that West Nile virus had arrived in New York City[5], far from its usual location.

Case reports are the first steps in discovering unexpected drug effects, both good and bad.[6] For example, sildenafil (Viagra) was developed initially as a treatment for angina, but a side effect observed in individual cases led to its marketing as a treatment for erectile dysfunction.[7]

Case reports led to the discovery of heart problems caused by drugs prescribed to suppress appetite[8], or muscle problems caused by contaminants in L-tryptophan.[9]

A well-written case report should provide clear evidence of the patient's problem or condition and its treatment. In addition, it should provide a clear explanation of why the reader should be surprised by the outcome of the case, with appropriate references.[10]

Clear evidence of the patient's initial problem or condition:

Because I work primarily with a nutritional therapy for cancer, I will use cancer as an illustration throughout this piece, though the principles can be applied to other illnesses. It is not uncommon to read patient testimonials that claim a diagnosis such as cancer was made, but do not provide evidence that cancer was present. For example, I have seen cases where a patient found a breast mass, was told by a doctor that it was "clearly cancer," refused surgical removal or biopsy, proceeded with some form of alternative therapy, and subsequently claimed miraculous cure.

The problem with this scenario is that cancer can only be diagnosed by a pathologist viewing a tissue sample under a microscope. It requires removal of tissue by biopsy or excision, or collection of samples for cytology. A doctor's clinical impression of cancer or a suspicious test result does not prove the presence of cancer.

As an example, in one study on the predictive ability of mammograms, lesions described as "highly predictive of malignancy" had an 81% chance of being found to be cancer when biopsy was performed—so 19% of the time, no cancer was present.[11]

In a case report, then, it should be clear exactly how the diagnosis was made. It should also be clear what treatment a patient might have received before embarking on the treatment that is being given credit for an unusual outcome.

Why the outcome is unusual:

For a case report to be worth reporting, the outcome of the patient in question must be remarkable or unusual in some way. In the case of cancer, unusual results can be prolonged survival, or stabilization, shrinkage or disappearance of the tumor mass. Cancer by its nature grows and spreads; stabilization over a prolonged period, shrinkage or disappearance are all unusual for a biopsy proven cancer.

To evaluate survival, the patient's case must be compared to a historical "control group" of the expected outcome of patients with their condition. For prolonged survival to be meaningful, it must extend well beyond the expected outcome—for example, if the usual prognosis is death five months after diagnosis, survival for six months is not impressive, but survival for 24 months is.

Expected outcome can be difficult for a layperson to assess, since they do not have the medical background to know what the usual outcome is for any given condition. A well written case history should describe the typical outcome, and the reference from which this information was obtained.

I have seen testimonials which state, "My doctor told me I would be dead within a year if I did not get the chemotherapy." This statement is the only evidence given that the outcome is unusual. Unfortunately, statements such as this may or may not be correct—patients may not hear what their doctor said correctly, or in some cases, the doctor may be overstating the benefits of chemotherapy.

For example, consider the following hypothetical scenarios:

A 60 year old woman has a lumpectomy and lymph node removal for breast cancer. She has a 1.5 cm tumor; the cancer has spread to two lymph nodes. She is told that she needs chemotherapy to prevent a recurrence. Her doctor tells her that "refusing chemotherapy is like committing suicide." She refuses and instead decides to pursue an alternative treatment. Ten years later, she is alive with no evidence of cancer.

Another woman has a lumpectomy and lymph node removal for breast cancer. She has two positive lymph nodes, receives chemotherapy, and one year later is found to have recurrent disease with tumors in the liver and brain. She refuses further chemotherapy, decides to pursue an alternative treatment, but has great difficulty in following it because of symptoms from her cancer. Three years after her diagnosis of metastatic disease, she dies.

Which outcome is unusual? In the first scenario, to assess her probable outcome after surgery, I went to the website Adjuvant! Online (http://www.adjuvantonline.com/index.jsp). This site provides information to help health professionals and patients with early stage cancer discuss the risks and benefits of getting additional therapy after the cancer has been surgically removed. This patient had a 52% chance of being alive and without evidence of cancer after 10 years with surgical treatment alone.[12] So her good outcome is not unusual. Had she gotten chemotherapy and hormone therapy, according to Adjuvant Online, her chances of being alive and without evidence of cancer in 10 years would have improved to 63%.

In the second hypothetical case, while review of the medical literature cannot answer precisely how long a patient with metastases to both the liver and brain might live, one article reports that breast cancer patients with metastatic disease to the brain have a median survival of 29 weeks (about 7 months).[13] In another study ofpatients with liver metastases from breast cancer, the median survival was 14 months.[14] In both cases, unlike our hypothetical patient, the study subjects received orthodox treatment for their illness. Even though the patient died, living three years with metastatic disease in the locations listed is unusual. Her case report is of interest, even though she died.

Limitations of case studies:

Case studies are good for picking up novelty, but they have limitations. Generally speaking, a case report cannot prove that the treatment described is actually what created or caused the desired result. And a case report cannot indicate if the experience described is typical; only statistical analysis of a larger treatment group, compared to a clearly defined control group, can do that. There are some situations where case reports are accepted as definitive evidence—a single case report can prove that a drug caused an adverse reaction.[15,16,17] The case report should include the following:

- Challenge—the reaction occurs when the drug is given
- De-challenge—the reaction resolves when the drug is stopped
- Re-challenge—the reaction recurs again when the drug is given

In the case of the treatment of disease, a similar scenario can create a stronger case report. For example, a patient under my colleague Dr. Gonzalez's care presented with metastatic breast cancer which resolved while she followed his recommendations, recurred when she quit, and resolved again when she resumed her nutritional protocol. This would argue that her nutritional protocol was effective against her disease.

Case reports can point more strongly to the treatment as the cause of the outcome when more than one is presented simultaneously. Sometimes individual cases of resolution of cancer are discounted as "spontaneous remissions." Spontaneous remissions, in the medical literature, refer to complete or partial resolution of cancer for no reason that the physician can discover or credit. Spontaneous remissions are not common. The author of a book[18] on spontaneous remission of cancer, Warren H. Cole, M.D., said in a 1974 interview: "The phenomenon is extremely rare. Some investigators estimate the incidence is as low as one in 100,000 cancer patients."[19] Given their rarity, it would be unusual for a single practitioner to see even one case of spontaneous remission during their career, let alone two or three. This would suggest that if an alternative practitioner can provide more than a few case reports with clear-cut unusual outcomes, there may be something worth investigating in that treatment.

The outcome described in a case report may not be the typical experience for patients pursuing a particular treatment. As an example, the drug Iressa created great excitement when it was first introduced for lung cancer, because some patients in initial case reports had amazing resolution of their disease.[20,21] The Food and Drug Administration approved it for use outside of research studies in May 2003 under its accelerated approval regulations. But when the drug was more extensively tested in controlled clinical trials, it was found that very few patients actually had any response.[22] Overall, there was no improvement in survival.[23]

Case reports as basis for further research:

Case reports ideally provide the basis for more definitive research. In studies such as randomized controlled trials, patients selected according to very specific criteria are assigned to treatment groups and followed prospectively. This can demonstrate whether the treatment is causing the desired effect, and show in what percentage of patients the desired effect is achieved. Clinical trials are relatively simple (though expensive) to implement in the case of a drug; for interventions such as dietary changes or frequent doses of nutritional supplements,problems with patient compliance can make it hard to generate useful information. Numerous studies have shown that patients tend to overestimate their compliance with medications[24] and dietary advice[25],or misrepresent it in an effort to gain the approval of the physician.[26] Because of the challenges of funding and of study design and implementation, very few trials of complementary or alternative therapies have been completed, and the results of almost all of those completed are debated.[27,28]

As a recent book on clinical case reporting states: "… because a case study is the first link in the chain of evidence, other steps do not necessarily have to follow for some time. A single case or case series (with all their inherent limitations) may long remain the only evidence available. If that happens, single cases or case series must provide the best evidence in their contexts."[29]

REFERENCES:

1. Doyle RP. The Medical Wars. William Morrow & Co., Inc., 1983.

2. Vandenbroucke JP. In defense of case reports. Ann Intern Med. 2001;134:330–334.

3. Gottlieb MS. Discovering AIDS. Epidemiology 1998;9:365–7.

4. Kolstoe J, Messner RP. Lyme disease: musculoskeletal manifestations. Rheum Dis Clin North Am. 1989;15:649–56.

5. Exotic diseases close to home. Lancet. 1999;354:1221

6. Bond RA. A proposal for a national program reporting beneficial drug responses, analogous to the existing program to detect adverse drug responses. Med Hypotheses. 2006;66:10–3.

7. Ghofrani HA, Osterloh IH, Grimminger F. Sildenafil: from angina to erectile dysfunction to pulmonary hypertension and beyond. Nat Rev Drug Discov. 2006;5:689–702.

8. Connolly HM, Crary JL, McGoon MD, Hensrud DD, Edwards BS, Edwards WD, Schaff HV. Valvular heart disease associated with fenfluramine-phentermine. N Engl J Med. 1997;337:581–8.

9. Hertzman PA, Blevins WL, Mayer J, Greenfield B, Ting M, Gleich GJ. Association of the eosinophilia-myalgia syndrome with the ingestion of tryptophan. N Engl J Med. 1990;322:869–73.

10. Vandenbroucke JP. Case reports in an evidence-based world. J R Soc Med. 1999;92:159–63.

11. Liberman L, Abramson AF, Squires FB, Glassman JR, Morris EA, Dershaw DD. The breast imaging reporting and data system: positive predictive value of mammographic features and final assessment categories. AJR Am J Roentgenol. 1998;171:35–40.

12. Adjuvant! for Breast Cancer (Version 8.0) at www.adjuvantonline.com. Accessed on September 27, 2006.

13. Lentzsch S, Reichardt P, Weber F, Budach V, Dorken B. Brain metastases in breast cancer: prognostic factors and management. Eur J Cancer. 1999;35:580–5.

14. Eichbaum MH, Kaltwasser M, Bruckner T, de Rossi TM, Schneeweiss A, Sohn C. Prognostic factors for patients with liver metastases from breast cancer. Breast Cancer Res Treat. 2006;96:53–62.

15. Calis KA, Young LR. Clinical analysis of adverse drug reactions. In: Atkinson AJ, Daniels CE, Dedrick RL, Grudzinskas CV, Markey SP, ed. Principles of Clinical Pharmacology. San Diego: Academic Press; 2001. p 327.

16. Ferrell GC. Drug-induced hepatic injury. J Gastroenterol Hepatol. 1997;12:S242–50

17. U.S. Food and Drug Administration Center for Biologics Evaluation and Research, April 2005. Guidance for industry: good pharmacovigilance practices and pharmacoepidemiologic assessment. Available at: http://www.fda.gov/cber/gdlns/pharmacovig.htm. Accessed on November 12, 2006.

18. Everson TC and Cole WH. Spontaneous Regression of Cancer. Philadelphia, WB Saunders Co., 1966.

19. Cole WH. Spontaneous regression of cancer. CA Cancer J Clin. 1974;24:274–9.

20. Fujiwara K, Kiura K, Ueoka H, Tabata M, Hamasaki S, Tanimoto M. Dramatic effect of ZD1839 ('Iressa') in a patient with advanced non-small-cell lung cancer and poor performance status. Lung Cancer. 2004;40:73–6.

21. Villano JL, Mauer AM, Vokes EE. A case study documenting the anticancer activity of ZD1839 (Iressa) in the brain. Ann Oncol. 2003;14:656–8.

22. US Food and Drug Administration Center for Drug Evaluation and Research. Questions and Answers on Iressa (gefitinib). http://www.fda.gov/cder/drug/infopage/iressa/iressaQ&A2005.htm. Accessed on November 12, 2006.

23. Thatcher N, Chang A, Parikh P, Rodrigues Pereira J, Ciuleanu T, von Pawel J, Thongprasert S, Tan EH, Pemberton K, Archer V, Carroll K. Gefitinib plus best supportive care in previously treated patients with refractory advanced non-small-cell lung cancer: results from a randomised, placebo-controlled, multicentre study (Iressa Survival Evaluation in Lung Cancer). Lancet. 2005; 366:1527–37.

24. Straka RJ, Fish JT, Benson SR, Suh JT. Patient self-reporting of compliance does not correspond with electronic monitoring: an evaluation using isosorbide dinitrate as a model drug. Pharmacotherapy. 1997;17:126–32

25. Kristal AR, Andrilla CH, Koepsell TD, Diehr PH, Cheadle A. Dietary assessment instruments are susceptible to intervention-associated response set bias. J Am Diet Assoc. 1998;98:40–3.

26. Hebert JR, Clemow L, Pbert L, Ockene IS, Ockene JK. Social desirability bias in dietary self-report may compromise the validity of dietary intake measures. Int J Epidemiol. 1995;24:389–98.

27. Lawvere S, Mahoney MC. St. John's wort. Am Fam Physician. 2005;72:2249–54.

28. Sood A, Sood R, Bauer BA, Ebbert JO. Cochrane systematic reviews in acupuncture: methodological diversity and database searching. J Altern Complement Med. 2005;11:719–22.

29. Jenicek M. Clinical Case Reporting In Evidence-Based Medicine; second edition. London: Arnold; 2001:58.

Remarks

By Mary McNair

While working as the Business Manager for Nicholas J. Gonzalez, MD, I had the privilege of watching him prepare for his pivotal NCI presentation in 1993. I remember the day he received the call to present—he was shocked and energized by the opportunity. He had worked so many years for a moment like this. We spoke of it every day leading up to the big day. "Nick" wanted so badly to represent the program in its truest, most authentic form. He wanted to get out of the way and let the success stories speak for themselves. He wanted me to pray for him, that he would have the courage to represent, not only the physical healing the program offered, but the relevance of the spiritual component necessary to succeed. He knew he needed a higher power greater than himself to intervene on his behalf.

The morning before he left for the NCI, Nick stopped by the office to check-in and pick up a few needed materials. He was nervous and sweating. It was obvious he took his mission very seriously and wanted to do a great job. After prompting him to fix his tie, I reminded him of the brilliance of his oratory skills and he laughed, eager to shake off the well-deserved compliments. I repeated to him again to be true to his original mission—to not water down the program and protocols he had prescribed to so many patients who had effectively followed it. As always, Nick's primary objective was to help save as many as possible from the diseases ravaging their bodies.

When he returned to the office from the NCI presentation, he was just as motivated and clear-headed as he had been the day he left. He wanted to squeeze just one more patient into his already-busy schedule.

Honestly, I have no idea the totality of the outcome from that visit. It did, however, illustrate to me one thing. Nick was all about his patients. He worked day and night, tirelessly, on their behalf. I have no doubt he would continue to do so if he were here today. My respect knows no bounds. He will forever be one of the greatest heroes in my life.

Mary McNair
Outer Cape Health Services
Director, Healthcare Center

Introduction
Presented to the National Cancer Institute, 1993

By Nicholas J. Gonzalez, M.D.

After completion of my second year at Cornell University Medical College in 1981, I had the opportunity to meet Dr. William Donald Kelley in New York. I had already known about Kelley, the Texas dentist who for twenty years had been treating cancer patients with a complicated nutritional therapy. At the time I met him, Dr. Kelley had achieved considerable notoriety because of his involvement in the case of Steve McQueen, the actor who died in late 1980 from advanced mesothelioma. Although Kelley had been repeatedly attacked in the press as an outright charlatan, the Dr. Kelley I met was an unassuming man whose primary wish was to have his controversial work fairly evaluated by the academic medical world. I thought his request reasonable.

My research advisor at Cornell agreed to support a case review of Kelley's patients, which I began intensively the summer of 1981, and continued despite the rigors of third year medical school. During my fourth year at Cornell, I was given a considerable block of time to investigate Kelley's work and results in a more structured manner. Eventually, what began as a student project developed into a two-year formal research effort that I pursued while an immunology fellow.

During my study, I reviewed nearly 10,000 of Dr. Kelley's patient records, which he kept divided between his Dallas and Washington State offices. I interviewed and evaluated intensively over 500 patients with appropriately diagnosed advanced cancer, and summarized my findings in an extended monograph completed in 1986 as partial fulfillment for my fellowship training.

The written report consisted of several sections. In addition to outlining Kelley's theoretical approach, I discussed at length 50 of his patients initially diagnosed with poor prognosis cancer, all of whom had enjoyed long term survival and/or apparent regression of disease while following their nutritional regimen. As a separate chapter, I also evaluated all patient cases of unresectable pancreatic cancer, both compliant and non-compliant, that had come to see Kelley between 1974 and 1982. I eventually identified 22 patients in this group. For all of these patients, I obtained complete medical records, including death certificates for those who were deceased. I interviewed all surviving patients repeatedly and at length, and in the case of those who had died, I interviewed family members as well as the original attending physicians.

Ten of these patients had visited Kelley only once and had never followed the protocol: these individuals had been discouraged from proceeding largely because of the influence of family and physicians who thought Kelley to be an outright fraud. This population, with a median survival of only 60 days, served as a convenient control. A second group of partial compliers consisted of seven patients who pursued the program incompletely, and for varying periods of time: again, family and physician pressure seemed to be the main reasons for their stopping the program.

Nonetheless, despite the incomplete compliance, the median survival for these patients was 300 days. A third group of five patients followed the program completely, and for this population the median survival, at the time I completed my study, was already over eight years. For patients with inoperable pancreatic cancer, such long-term survival was something I had not expected.

Despite the careful documentation and the five-year investment of time, my attempts at publication were met with scorn and ridicule. It seemed no one in academic medicine could, at the time, accept that a nutritional therapy might produce such positive results with advanced cancer patients. Of course, Kelley's own dubious reputation didn't help my publishing efforts.

In 1986, probably as a result of endless pressures, Kelley suffered what amounts to a psychotic break. Since that time, he has been living largely as a hermit, writing and publishing bizarre political tracts. He has long given up any research or patient care, and I myself have not spoken to him since 1987. In that year, I decided to move to New York to try and salvage Kelley's treatment, and observe for myself the results with poor prognosis cancer patients. Now, after six years, I have found the treatment effective with patients suffering poor prognosis or evident terminal disease. Twenty-five of these patients are described in the accompanying report.

The therapy itself is quite complex, but basically involves three components: **diet, aggressive supplementation with nutrients and enzymes, and detoxification**. I have my own method of evaluating patients, largely based on Kelley's system, and the protocols are individualized. Each patient on The Gonzalez Protocol receives a diet designed for his or her specific needs, and the diets are quite variable, ranging from a pure vegetarian "nuts and seeds" program to a diet requiring fatty red meat 2–3 times a day.

The supplement regimens are also individualized, and intense: each cancer patient consumes between 130 and 160 capsules daily. The supplement programs include a range of vitamins, minerals and trace elements, prescribed according to the particular patient's needs and cancer type. These nutrients do not, I believe, have a direct anti-cancer effect, but instead serve to improve overall metabolic function.

In addition to nutrients, every patient takes large quantities of freeze-dried porcine pancreatic enzymes in capsule form, which provide the main anti-cancer action. Kelley believed, as do I, that the circulating pancreatic proteolytic enzymes provide a direct and powerful anti-tumor activity. Kelley was not the first to propose such an effect for the enzymes: Dr. John Beard, an eminent Scottish embryologist, first suggested in 1904 that the pancreas and its enzymes are the body's main defense against cancer. In 1911, Dr. Beard published a monograph entitled *The Enzyme Therapy of Cancer* (published by New Spring Press in X), which summarized his theory and the supporting evidence.

After Beard presented his thesis, a number of case reports appeared in the mainstream medical literature documenting tumor regression and even "cure" in a number of terminal cancer patients treated with only injectable pancreatic enzymes. However, after Beard's death around 1915, his work was largely forgotten until resurrected by Kelley in the early 1960's.

Basic science support for this work does exist: in 1965 two articles appeared in the mainstream literature documenting a significant anti-cancer effect for the enzymes in a tumor prone animal model. Leighton King, a researcher at St. Joseph's Hospital in Arizona, reported complete prevention of tumors in a group of C3H mice carrying Bittner's milk factor virus who received oral pancreatin, compared to 100% tumor occurrence in the control group (King, Leighton: "Prevention of Virus-Induced Mammary Tumors by an Orally Active Pancreas Factor," Experimental Medicine and Surgery, Vol 25, No. 4, pp. 345–347, December 1965). In a second article, King proposed an immune enhancement effect for orally ingested pancreatin; in an experimental group of Swiss mice, he described a 260% increase in antibody production with the addition of 2% pancreatin to the diet (King, Leighton: "A Novel Method of Enhancing Antibody Production," Southwestern Medicine, Vol 36, No. 7, July 1965). Although these results seem impressive, this research never received the attention I believe it deserved.

The actual mechanism of action for the enzyme effect has not been described. I suspect the proteolytic proteins have a direct anti-cancer capability, as well as indirect activity mediated via immune enhancement. Whatever the pathway, normal tissues seem completely unaffected. Furthermore, although most scientists in my personal experience believe orally ingested enzymes will be degraded in the gut, King's animal work—and the experience of Kelley and myself— indicates otherwise. The enzymes, when consumed in their inactive form, survive destruction in the stomach and in turn are activated and absorbed in the alkaline small intestine.

The third component of the protocol, detoxification, generally evokes the greatest scorn among orthodox oncologists. Kelley believed that as the enzymes attack a tumor and as a damaged body repairs, significant amounts of toxic wastes accumulate: these waste products could, he maintained, provoke a variety of symptoms ranging from high fever and headaches to palpitations and arthritis. Kelley incorporated a variety of techniques into his program, including coffee enemas, to aid liver function and speed up efficient handling of these toxic by-products.

During my investigation of Kelley's work, I was surprised to uncover a rich literature from the 1920's and 1930's detailing, in the orthodox journals, the therapeutic value of enemas. For example, a study from Lenox Hill Hospital published in 1929 demonstrated gallbladder emptying, believed stimulated through autonomic reflexes, after the rectal instillation of a variety of materials.

Of the hundreds of Kelley patients I interviewed during my research study, virtually every one reported significant symptomatic relief from the enemas. In my own practice patients repeatedly report the same improved well-being and relief of symptoms after a coffee enema. I suspect the enemas initiate a parasympathetic response that in turn feeds back to the liver and causes a release of stored wastes. And despite the frequent dangers attributed to coffee enemas, I have yet to d ocument a single serious side effect either in the thousands of Kelley patients I evaluated, or in my own practice. I have patients who have routinely done up to 12 coffee enemas day without electrolyte disturbances or other problems: the only side effect reported is that the patients "feel better."

In the following section, I present 25 case reports selected from among my own patients. The great majority of these people presented with poor prognosis or terminal disease, and for most I provide evidence for reduction of tumor mass. In several cases, I document unusual tumor stabilization for periods of years, though not outright regression of disease.

For all but one patient, I provide appropriate tissue diagnosis. The exception is a woman with a presumed diagnosis, based on CT studies, of pancreatic cancer but with no histological documentation: although I realize this case cannot be considered definitive, I decided to include her story nonetheless because I find her history, and her radiographically documented improvement, informative.

Breast Cancer

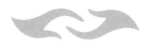

1. Patient: AF
DOB: 10/9/24

Patient AF is a 68 year-old white female nurse with a history of metastatic breast cancer. In July 1987, she first noticed a left breast mass. Her physician referred her for mammography, which showed a suspicious lesion. After a needle biopsy confirmed carcinoma, patient AF underwent a modified radical mastectomy at Mercy San Juan Hospital; the pathology report describes mixed colloid carcinoma and intraductal and infiltrating duct carcinoma, with 1/7 nodes positive for malignancy. However, a subsequent metastatic work-up was negative. When estrogen receptor studies were positive, she was started on tamoxifen.

Patient AF did well until September 1988 when a routine CEA was elevated at 14. CT scan showed multiple new tumors in the liver, consistent with metastatic disease. A bone scan and a chest X-ray were both negative for metastatic disease.

In November 1988, patient AF began CMF chemotherapy. After six cycles of chemotherapy, a repeat CT scan showed no improvement, and her oncologist added vincristine to her protocol in May 1989. However, she suffered such severe side effects that she decided, with her oncologist's support, to discontinue chemotherapy. She was told that her survival would most likely be measured in months.

Patient AF heard about my therapy and came to see me for the first time on June 26, 1989. At that time, examination was notable only for evidence of prior mastectomy and evidence of a mild peripheral neuropathy. After patient AF returned to California to begin her protocol, her local oncologist sent her for a baseline abdominal CT scan which revealed that the liver tumors had only progressed despite chemotherapy, as documented in the official report:

"There are several low attenuation lesions about the liver, the largest measuring 3 cm. in the lateral segment of the left lobe of the liver. This lesion appears enlarged since the prior examination. Additionally, a new lesion is noted about the right lobe of the liver. These likely represent metastatic disease."

Patient AF initially suffered ups and downs on her nutritional protocol, but she remained compliant and determined. Her local oncologist in California continued to follow her progress, and after she had completed nearly a year on her protocol, a CT scan of the abdomen on April 3, 1990 revealed significant improvement as documented in the written report:

"Comparison is made to the prior examination on 7/12/89. Since then, the metastatic lesions in the liver have decreased slightly in size. The low attenuation lesion in the medial segment of the left lobe now measures 2 cm in diameter as compared to 3 cm on the previous examination. That in the anterior segment of the right lobe now measures 2 cm as compared to previous measurement of 2.5 cm in diameter. No new lesions are identified."

Patient AF continued on her nutritional protocol and on April 15, 1991, nearly two years after beginning her program, she went for another CT scan that again revealed improvement:

"Multiple small liver lesions most of which measure less than 5 mm in diameter in the medial segment of left lobe as well as anterior and posterior segments of right lobe." Then, when patient AF completed three years on her protocol, a follow-up CT scan done June 4, 1992 showed that the largest tumor, which previously had been solid, now appeared to be cystic:

"1. Three hypodense hepatic lesions remaining, the largest of which is located in the posterior segment of the right lobe of the liver, measuring approximately 1 cm in diameter, and has the CT characteristics of a simple cyst. The other hepatic lesions are smaller on the current study compared with the prior study (of 4/5/91). 2. No evidence of retroperitoneal adenopathy."

Today, patient AF has completed over four years on her nutritional protocol, and generally appears to be in excellent health.

Dr. Gonzalez presented these 25 cancer case studies to the NCI in 1993 and then updated the patient status information in 2001. Below are Dr. Gonzalez's personal notes with updated survival information:

Metastatic breast cancer. Quit the program after over 4 years and eventually died.

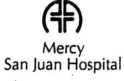

Mercy San Juan Hospital

TISSUE EXAMINATION

RECEIVED JUL   198

PATIENT:
HOSP. L NO: 3.   AGE 62
ROOM NO: JULY , 198
DATE
DOCTOR(S):   ⌐. REED, MD

ACCESSION NO: S-   -8

Preoperative diagnosis: Left breast mass
Postoperative diagnosis: Same

EXAMINATION OF TISSUE FROM LEFT BREAST BIOPSY

GROSS DESCRIPTION
A. Specimen received fresh labeled "left breast biopsy" consists of gray-pink fragments of fatty pieces of tissue, approximately 0.8 x 0.6 x 0.4 cm. Frozen section diagnosis "colloid carcinoma--material set aside for ERA/PRA. Additional to come from mastectomy specimen"/LML. Small amount of remaining tissue submitted in one cassette.

B. Specimen received fresh consists of a mastectomy with axillary dissection. Additional tumor removed and frozen for estrogen and progesterone receptor assay. The specimen measures about 25 x 17 x 3 cm overall and contains a 21 x 5.5 cm skin ellipse with an eccetrically placed nipple and areola. A recent sutured surgical incision is present lateral to the areola. The undersurface shows fascia with focal muscle fibers. The attached axillary dissection by 5 x 2 cm and contains palpable nodes. Most of the breast tissue is atrophic, with residual fibrous tissue around the areola showing ductectasia. The remaining tumor measures 3 x 3 x approximately 1.5 cm and is present at the deep level of the breast adjacent to the fascia. It is well demarcated from the remainder of the breast and has a firm fleshy appearance. The tumor is translucent, tan with white opaque fibrous streaks. The margins are scalloped. The axillary dissection is arbitrarily divided into low, middle and upper thirds. The lowest third contains 3 apparent lymph nodes ranging from 1 to 2 cm in maximum dimension. On sectioning they are quite fatty, without suspicion of metastasis. Representative sections submitted in one cassette. The mid axillary portion contains 2 lymph nodes, the larger one showing extensive fatty replacement and the smaller one, which measures about 1 cm, showing focal tumor metastasis in a subcapsular distribution. Representative sections submitted in one cassette. The upper axillary portion contains 2 possible lymph nodes measuring about 1 and 1.5 cm in diameter. These show fatty replacement without sign of metastasis and are submitted in one cassette. JLD:jla

- CONTINUED -

DEPARTMENT OF LABORATORY MEDICINE
MERCY SAN JUAN HOSPITAL
CARMICHAEL, CALIFORNIA

_____ M.D.

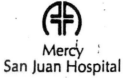

**Mercy
San Juan Hospital**

TISSUE EXAMINATION

PATIENT:
HOS...AL NO: 3..   AGE 62
ROOM NO: JULY ., 198
DATE   J. REED, MD
DOCTOR(S):

ACCESSION NO: S- -8

Page Two

MICROSCOPIC DESCRIPTION
A. Sections are of breast tissue in which there is a colloid
carcinoma present. Small and large nests of relatively uniform
epithelial cells are floating in pools of mucin. The adjacent
breast tissue shows fibrocystic disease.

B. Sections taken of the tumor in the mastectomy specimen show
similar areas of abundant mucin production. In addition to this,
however, there are areas of conventional intraductal and invasive
duct carcinoma. The mucinous component comprises the majority.
Tumor is observed in numerous lymphatic spaces outside the main
tumor mass. The adjacent breast tissue shows fibrocystic disease
of the proliferative type. Sections taken of the nipple show no
evidence of Paget's disease and no involvement of superficial
ducts or lymphatics by tumor. Sections of the submitted lymph
nodes show a single positive node in the mid axilla. The entire
node is replaced by tumor which resembles the primary, with
predominant mucin production.

DIAGNOSIS: A,B. Left breast biopsy and left mastectomy
                     with axillary dissection:
                     1. Mixed colloid (mucinous) carcinoma and
                         intraductal and infiltrating duct
                         carcinoma
                     2. One of seven left axillary lymph nodes,
                         positive for metastatic adenocarcinoma
                     3. Fibrocystic disease, proliferative type

(1)

Coded (R)

ELL:llr
7- -8

DEPARTMENT OF LABORATORY MEDICINE
MERCY SAN JUAN HOSPITAL
CARMICHAEL, CALIFORNIA

_____ M.D.

Emily L. Leff, M.D>

Mercy San Juan Hospital

DEPARTMENT OF RADIOLOGY

```
PATIENT:      A  _ F
M.R.#:
ORDER #:      1448216
ACCOUNT #:
ROOM #:
D.O.B.:        / /24
PHYSICIAN:    J. KAILATH, M.D.
TYPE:         OP
CC:           J. REED
              W. MATTHEWS
```

DATE: 4/3/90
PROCEDURE: CT SCAN OF THE ABDOMEN

Scanning was performed through the abdomen following oral and intravenous contrast administration.

FINDINGS: Comparison is made to the prior examination on 7/12/89. Since then, the metastatic lesions in the liver have decreased slightly in size. The low attenuation lesion in the medial segment of the left lobe now measures 2 cm in diameter as compared to 3 cm on the previous examination. That in the anterior segment of the right lobe measures 2 cm as compared to previous measurement of 2.5 cm in diameter. No new lesions are identified. The pancreas and kidneys remain normal in appearance. The spleen is normal as well. There is no evidence of retroperitoneal adenopathy.

IMPRESSION: SLIGHT DECREASE IN SIZE OF METASTATIC LESIONS IN THE LIVER
                   AS DISCUSSED.

                              PETER L. JAMES, M.D.

PLJ/TC:kc
D: 4/3/90
T: 4/3/90
Doc #: 3344x-3
Code #: 197.7

6501 Coyle Avenue
Carmichael, CA 95608
(916) 537-5000

A Division of Catholic Healthcare West

Mercy Healthcare Sacramento **Nuclear Medicine Report**

MERCY SAN JUAN HOSPITAL

```
PATIENT:      A    F
MED. REC.:
SCAN:         4131-90
SEX:          F    AGE:  66
ROOM NO:      OP
PHYSICIAN:    JOHN KAILATH, M.D.

              Document:  1627B
```

Copy to Dr. Wayne Matthews

PROCEDURE: WHOLE BODY BONE SCAN

DATE: 11/13/90

RADIOPHARMACEUTICAL: Tc 99m MDP   DOSE: 19.3 mCi

CLINICAL INDICATION:
Breast cancer, low back pain, evaluate for skeletal metastasis.

RESULTS:
No evidence of skeletal metastasis.

FINDINGS:
Following the intravenous administration of Tc 99m MDP, anterior and posterior whole body images and detailed spot views of the spine, bony thorax, and pelvis including the hips were obtained. Spinal labeling is mildly inhomogeneous and associated with loss of normal bony detail. There is low grade focal accentuation at the cervicothoracic junction to the left of midline, within a thoracic vertebra at approximately T4, and within the mid lumbar region most notable anteriorly. No dominant focal abnormalities are noted within the spine and, likewise, the remainder of the visualized skeletal structures are devoid of any dominant focal abnormality of a nonarticular nature.

The appendicular skeleton demonstrates low grade areas of increased periarticular labeling about the shoulders, right hand and wrist. The skeletal structures are elsewhere unremarkable. The renal silhouettes appear normal in size and position, there is no evidence of obstruction to urinary flow.

COMMENT:
This examination is devoid of any dominant focal abnormality of a nonarticular nature to suggest that the patient has developed skeletal metatasis from her underlying carcinoma of the breast. Comparison is made with the patient's last similar examination performed in October 1988. The only substantive interval change is the apparent resolution of an inferior right rib lesion supporting the impression at that time that this represented a benign change. Changes involving the axial and appendicular skeleton described above are abnormal but felt to be most consistent with benign osteoarthritic disease.

_____,M.D.
              Herman Kensky, M.D.

HK/sg   D&T: 11/13/90   198.5

Form # 25622

Mercy Healthcare Sacramento   Imaging Services Report

MERCY SAN JUAN HOSPITAL
6501 Coyle Ave.
Carmichael, California 95608
Phone (916)537-5191

PATIENT: A   F
MED. REC.:
ORDER: 1962887
ACCOUNT:
ROOM NO:
TYPE: OP
D.O.B.:   10/9/24
PHYSICIAN: JOHN KAILATH,M.D.

Document: 0682C

(handwritten: Copy to Dr. ...)

DATE: 4/15/91
PROCEDURE: CT OF THE ABDOMEN

TECHNIQUE:
Following oral contrast administration and during intravenous contrast dynamic
infusion, contiguous axial 10 mm scans of the abdomen were obtained from the
dome of the diaphragm to the iliac crest. The patient's previous CT studies
have been sent to Dr. Reed and are presently not available for comparison.
When old films do become available, an addendum to this report may be made.
Comparison was made with previous report of a CT scan performed on April 3,
1990.

FINDINGS:
The liver and spleen remain of normal size. Several small discrete lesions
measuring less than 5 mm in diameter are noted in the medial segment of the
left lobe as well as in the anterior and posterior segments of the right
lobe. Comparison with the previous report suggests that these lesions have
further decreased in size but again, once the old films become available, an
addendum to this report may be made. There are no large lesions visible. The
adrenal glands, spleen, pancreas and kidneys all remain of normal size and
have a normal pattern of enhancement without focal mass lesions. In the
retroperitoneum, there is no pathological adenopathy. Incidental note was
made that there is patchy sclerosis of the vertebral bodies of the lumbar
spine. Although some of these changes may be degenerative, if clinically
indicated, correlation with bone scan is suggested to exclude the possibility
of bony metastasis. Incidental note is also made that the wall of the stomach
appears mildly thickened, however, this may partly be due to partial volume
averaging of a partially distended stomach. Again, review of the patient's
past CT scans may be helpful to clarify this.

CONCLUSION:
1.   Multiple small liver lesions most of which measure less than 5 mm in
      diameter in medial segment of left lobe as well as anterior and posterior
      segments of the right lobe. Comparison with the previous report suggests
      that the lesions have further decreased in size.
2.   Patchy areas of sclerosis in the vertebral bodies. Although these are
      near the end-plates and may be related to degenerative change, we would
      suggest correlating with bone scan to rule out the possibility of bony
      metastasis.

FORM # 15008

Mercy Healthcare Sacramento   **Imaging Services Report**

MERCY SAN JUAN HOSPITAL
6501 Coyle Ave.
Carmichael, California 95608
Phone (916)537-5191

PATIENT:	A R F
MED. REC.:	
ORDER:	1962887
ACCOUNT:	
ROOM NO:	
TYPE:	OP
D.O.B.:	10/9/24
PHYSICIAN:	JOHN KAILATH,M.D.

3.   Stomach wall thickening in the fundus. This is probably partial volume
     averaging of partly distended stomach. Again review of the patient's
     past CTs could be helpful for further evaluation.

                              MIGUEL NIEVES, M.D.

MN:sg
D: 4/15/91
T: 4/15/91
Code #: 174.9

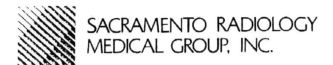

SACRAMENTO RADIOLOGY MEDICAL GROUP, INC.

Diagnostic Imaging Consultation Report

San Juan Plaza
6660 Coyle Avenue, Suite 200
Carmichael, California 95608

(916) 965-1913 • Fax (916) 863-1218

```
A    , F.                                      ALLEN PRIEST JR M.D.
                                               7529 SUNSET AVENUE
CERVICAL SPINE COMP          05/01/92          FAIR OAKS CA 95628
D.O.B.:        /24
```

FINDINGS: The patient is osteoporotic. The cervical vertebral bodies are intact. There is straightening of the cervical curvature. There is disc space narrowing at C4-5 and C5-6. There are degenerative changes from C3 to C7. Posterior elements are intact. The neural foramina are patent. There is mild narrowing of the right C4-5 and C5-6 neural foramina.

CONCLUSION:

Degenerative changes of the cervical spine.

Theresa De Marco, MD

TD/bjs-06   078074
                                                                 adge01
dc: 723

Mercy Healthcare Sacramento

Imaging Services Report

MERCY SAN JUAN HOSPITAL
Diagnostic Imaging Services
6501 Coyle Ave.
Carmichael, California 95608
Phone (916)537-5191

PATIENT: A . F .
MED. REC.:
ORDER: 2606309
ACCOUNT:
ROOM NO:
TYPE: OP
D.O.B.:   24
PHYSICIAN: John M. Kaliath, M.D.
              Wayne Matthews, M.D.
              John M. Reed, M.D.

              Document: 01235

DATE: 06/04/92
PROCEDURE: ABDOMINAL CT

Comparison is made with prior examination of 4/15/91.

TECHNIQUE:
Contiguous thinly collimated transaxial images were obtained through the abdomen following oral and intravenous contrast. 150 cc of Conray 60 was given without incident.

FINDINGS:
Several small hepatic hypodense lesions are demonstrated, the largest and most discreet of which is located in the posterior segment of the right lobe of the liver and has relatively sharp margins and density similar to that of water, consistent with a simple cyst. It appears slightly larger than on the prior study, however there are differences in the level of the sections obtained, and this is really only visualized on two images, thus making partial volume averaging artifact the most likely explanation for the inaterval change in size. The next most discrete lesion is very ill defined and located in the medial segment of the left lobe of the liver, and is less discrete than on the prior study. The previously described largest lesion noted in the anterior segment of the right lobe of the liver laterally is no longer well visualized, however is still barely discernible on the liver windows and is clearly smaller in size. No gallstones are demonstrated. The pancreas is unremarkable. The spleen is normal. No retroperitoneal lymphadenopathy is present. The adrenals and kidneys are normal.

IMPRESSION:
1.   Three hypodense hepatic lesions remaining, the largest of which is located in the posterior segment of the right lobe of the liver, measuring approximately 1 cm in greatest dimension, and has the CT characteristics of a simple cyst. The other hepatic lesions are smaller on the current study compared with the prior study.
2.   No evidence of retroperitoneal adenopathy.

                        ROLAND D. DEMARCO, M.D.

RDD:tg
D: 06/04/92 @1530 pu
T: 06/04/92 @1553
Code #: 197.7

RM #15008

2. Patient: JB
DOB: 5/1/40

Patient JB is a 53 year-old white woman with a history of recurrent chest wall breast cancer. Patient JB had been previously in good health when in 1985 she first noted a left breast mass. After refusing any type of standard intervention for what was thought to be a suspicious lesion, she eventually consented to surgery in 1988 after the lesion began to rapidly enlarge. On May 5, 1988 at the Evergreen Hospital Medical Center in Washington, she underwent a modified radical mastectomy for what was found to be infiltrating carcinoma. The primary tumor was quite large at 8 × 5 cm. and 8/15 axillary nodes were positive for metastatic disease.

Patient JB refused the recommended chemotherapy and radiation, and instead pursued treatment with Cancell. However, in early 1989, while on Cancell, she developed a chest wall recurrence that was biopsied on May 5, 1989 and found to be recurrent carcinoma. A metastatic work-up including bone scan, chest X-ray and CT scan, was negative.

Because of her worsening disease, patient JB decided to pursue my therapy and was initially seen in my office on January 31, 1990. At that time, she felt well and had no complaints aside from the lesions on the chest wall. She was taking tamoxifen 10 mg twice daily, but felt the lesions had been progressing despite the medication. Her examination was notable for half a dozen 1–2 cm. nodular lesions on her chest wall overlying the mastectomy site.

Upon returning home to Seattle, patient JB discontinued tamoxifen and began her nutritional protocol. She has been a very compliant patient over the past 3.5 years, remains dedicated to her protocol, and is in "excellent" general health. Her chest wall lesions initially stabilized and at present are scabbing over and regressing. Progress has been slow, but definite. She has been followed by a local oncologist in Seattle, but has received no other treatment other than mine since 1990.

Clearly, patient JB is an interesting patient. Both the size of her tumor and the eight positive axillary nodes at the time of surgery in May of 1988 indicated a very poor prognosis situation, further worsened by the chest wall recurrence. However, on her nutritional protocol her chest lesions, and her general health, have improved.

Dr. Gonzalez presented these 25 cancer case studies to the NCI in 1993 and then updated the patient status information in 2001. Below are Dr. Gonzalez's personal notes with updated survival information:

Metastatic breast cancer. Quit the program after nearly 5 years. I understand she is still alive although not disease free.

	J B.		DATE OF BIRTH 5-1-40	LAB. NUMBER	PAS CODE

PAS CODE
1 - Not abnormal
2 - Abn other than below
3 - Mechanical abn
4 - Growth alteration
5 - Degeneration & necrosis
6 - Nonacute inflam
7 - Acute inflam
8 - Nonmalig neoplasm
9 - Malignant neoplasm

PHYSICIAN: DeShazo - Evergreen Surgical Clinic (E051)

DATE: 5-13-88

SPECIMEN OF: Left breast needle biopsies.

Previous pathology: 87T4211-9, 3-20-87
DX: Needle biopsy, left breast with fibrous stroma and sclerosing adenosis, benign.

MACROSCOPIC: The specimen consists of two strips of tissue from a needle biopsy. Frozen section diagnosis: Carcinoma, (H. Siimo, M.D.). All is submitted.
HS/bm 5-13-88

MICROSCOPIC: Sections are through strips of breast tissue from needle biopsy showing areas of infiltrating strands and clusters of tumor cells with scant, poorly defined cytoplasm and moderately pleomorphic nuclei. The stroma is dense and desmoplastic. Very little normal mammary tissue is identified.
HS/pm 5-16-88

DIAGNOSIS: LEFT BREAST NEEDLE BIOPSY: INFILTRATING DESMOPLASTIC CARCINOMA.

Signed By _____ M.D.

Reported By _____ M.D.
Helju Siimo, M.D.

PSIP PUGET SOUND INSTITUTE OF PATHOLOGY

P.O. Box 21127, SEATTLE, WA 98111
(206) 622-4330/1-800-542-0702 OUT OF STATE WATTS 1-800-327-2712

Alex A. Ritzen, M.D.   Robert D. Hoag, M.D.
Charles E. Salzer, M.D.   M. Jane Mutti, M.D.
Helju Siimo, M.D.   Roger W. Graham, M.D.

PATHOLOGY REPORT

	. B	#21 12 72	-40		
PHYSICIAN	C. Deshazo - Evergreen General Hospital (E010)			DATE 5-25-88	4 - Growth alteration 5 - Degeneration & necrosis
SPECIMEN OF	A. Left breast. B. Biopsy, right breast.				6 - Nonacute inflam 7 - Acute inflam 8 - Nonmalig neoplasm 9 - Malignant neoplasm

Previous pathology: 87T4211-9, 3-20-87,
DX: Needle biopsy left breast with fibrous
stroma and sclerosing adenosis, benign.
88T7227-2, 5-13-88, Left breast needle
biopsy: infiltrating desmoplastic
carcinoma.

CLINICAL INFORMATION: Carcinoma, left breast.

MACROSCOPIC: A. Received is a left mastectomy measuring 15 x 12 x 6.5
cm. Attached is a 14 x 6 cm. ellipse of skin with a centrally placed
nipple. Attached is an 8.0 x 3.5 x 1.5 cm. axillary tail. Beneath the
nipple, within the main portion of the mastectomy is a very large carcinoma
which involves most of the breast parenchyma. The greatest dimensions of
this tumor are 8.0 x 5.0 cm. The lateral and deep margins of the
mastectomy, however, are widely free of involvement by tumor. The tumor
appears confluent and relatively well circumscribed. Tissue is removed for
estrogen receptor assay. Multiple representative sections are submitted.

B. A 5.5 x 3.0 cm. fibrofatty breast biopsy which shows some evidence of
fibrocystic change grossly. Frozen section diagnosis: Benign breast
parenchyma (M. Mauney, M.D.). Representative sections submitted.
MM/hb 5-25-88

MICROSCOPIC: A. Sections of the left breast show extensive invasion by
poorly differentiated adenocarcinoma which often invades in an Indian-file
fashion. The tumor is often signet ring cell in morphology. Occasionally
glands are formed. Features of both lobular and ductal carcinoma are
expressed. Sections of nipple are unremarkable. 8 of 15 axillary lymph
nodes contain metastatic carcinoma.

B. Sections show mild fibrocystic changes and a focus of atypical lobular
hyperplasia characterized by filling and expansion of lobules by small
uniform cells. This process only involves one lobule and complete
obliteration of lobular architecture is not appreciated.
MM/as 5-27-88

(continued on page 2)

Signed By_____ M.D.

Reported By_____ M.D.

 PUGET SOUND INSTITUTE OF PATHOLOGY

P.O. Box 21127, SEATTLE, WA 98111
(206) 622-4330/1-800-542-0702 OUT OF STATE WATTS 1-800-327-2712

Alex A. Ritzen, M.D.   Robert D. Hoag, M.D.
Charles E. Salzer, M.D.   M. Jane Mutti, M.D.
Helju Siimo, M.D.   Roger W. Graham, M.D.

PATHOLOGY REPORT

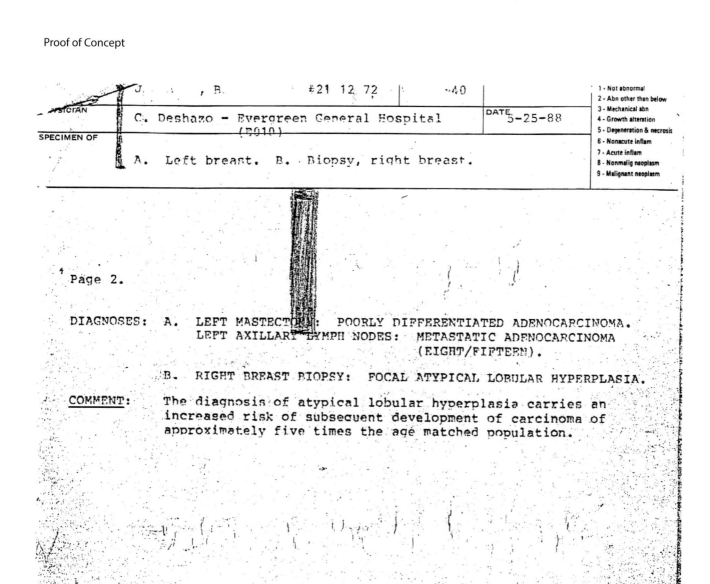

J.   , B.   #21 12 72 | ~40

	1 - Not abnormal
	2 - Abn other than below
	3 - Mechanical abn
	4 - Growth alteration
	5 - Degeneration & necrosis
	6 - Nonacute inflam
	7 - Acute inflam
	8 - Nonmalig neoplasm
	9 - Malignant neoplasm

C. Deshazo – Evergreen General Hospital   DATE 5-25-88
(B010)

SPECIMEN OF

A. Left breast. B. Biopsy, right breast.

Page 2.

DIAGNOSES: A.   LEFT MASTECTOMY: POORLY DIFFERENTIATED ADENOCARCINOMA.
             LEFT AXILLARY LYMPH NODES: METASTATIC ADENOCARCINOMA
                                   (EIGHT/FIFTEEN).

             B.   RIGHT BREAST BIOPSY: FOCAL ATYPICAL LOBULAR HYPERPLASIA.

COMMENT: The diagnosis of atypical lobular hyperplasia carries an
             increased risk of subsequent development of carcinoma of
             approximately five times the age matched population.

Signed By _____ M.D.

Reported By _____ Marc Mauney, M.D. _____ M.D.

PSIP PUGET SOUND INSTITUTE OF PATHOLOGY

P.O. Box 21127, SEATTLE, WA 98111
(206) 622-4330/1-800-542-0702 OUT OF STATE WATTS 1-800-327-2712

Alex A. Ritzen, M.D.   Robert D. Hoag, M.D.
Charles E. Salzer, M.D.   M. Jane Mutti, M.D.
Helju Siimo, M.D.   Roger W. Graham, M.D.

PATHOLOGY REPORT

			DATE OF BIRTH	LAB. NUMBER	PAS CODE
	J B.				1 - Not abnormal 2 - Abn other than below 3 - Mechanical abn 4 - Growth alteration 5 - Degeneration & necrosis 6 - Nonacute inflam 7 - Acute inflam 8 - Nonmalig neoplasm 9 - Malignant neoplasm
PHYSICIAN	DeShazo - Evergreen Surgical Clinic (E051)			DATE 5-5-89	
SPECIMEN OF	Excision lesion of chest.				

MACROSCOPIC: Submitted is an elliptical portion of skin 7 x 5 mm. Surface is smooth and glistening. The surgical margins are marked with blue ink and the specimen is bisected and totally embedded.
CES/mg 5-7-89

MICROSCOPIC: The sections reveal skin showing in the dermal collagen infiltrating poorly differentiated adenocarcinoma. The tumor is present as relatively small cells with enlarged irregular shaped nuclei, varying amounts of cytoplasm and arranged in strands and small nests of tumor in the stroma. The border is infiltrating and there is no evidence of circumscription.
AAR/as 5-8-89

DIAGNOSIS: SKIN OF CHEST SHOWING CARCINOMA CONSISTENT WITH BREAST PRIMARY.

COMMENT: Review of the previous tissue #88T7866 reveals cells with
             similar morphologic pattern metastatic to the lymph nodes.

Signed By _____ M.D.

Reported By _____ M.D.
            Alex A. Ritzen, M.D.

PSIP PUGET SOUND INSTITUTE OF PATHOLOGY

P.O. Box 21145 SEATTLE, WA 98111
(206) 448-7747/1-800-542-0702 OUT OF STATE WATTS 1-800-327-2712

Alex A. Ritzen, M.D.   M. Jane Mutti, M.D.
Charles E. Salzer, M.D.   Roger W. Graham, M.D.
Robert D. Hoag, M.D.   Helju Siimo, M.D.
            Marc Mauney, M.D.

3. Patient: LJ
DOB: 6/16/42

Patient LJ is a 50 year-old white female psychotherapist with a history of widely metastatic breast cancer. Patient LJ has a strong family history of breast cancer, but had previously been in good health when in October of 1986, routine mammography demonstrated a suspicious mass in the left breast. Biopsy of the lesion on October 30, 1986 revealed ductal carcinoma in situ. Although her surgeon suggested a modified radical mastectomy, patient LJ insisted only on a lumpectomy, which was done in early November at St. Luke's Hospital, Denver. The pathology report confirms carcinoma. At that time, there was no evidence of metastatic disease and she received no additional treatment.

Patient LJ subsequently did well until July of 1989, when her physician detected a mass in the right breast. A lumpectomy on July 7, 1989 documented poorly differentiated adenocarcinoma and a resected 3 cm. axillary node was partially replaced by metastatic tumor. Abdominal ultrasound revealed a density on the right lobe of the liver consistent with metastatic disease, and a needle biopsy on July 24, 1989 confirmed carcinoma. A bone scan showed increased uptake at C5 thought due to degenerative disease.

Patient LJ then began chemotherapy with CAF, which she tolerated poorly. In November of 1989, after completing three cycles, she refused further treatment. For several months, she did nothing, but in March 1990, she went to Stanford for an additional opinion. There, the physicians reviewed her previous studies and scans and concurred with the diagnosis of metastatic disease to the liver. Her doctor at Stanford recommended she immediately resume chemotherapy with CMF. But again, patient LJ refused to consider further orthodox therapy, and instead, after learning of my work, decided to pursue my program. She was first seen in my office on April 19, 1990. At that time, she reported feeling tired, and reported significant "liver pain" that at times was disabling. She also reported a new right breast mass. She was on no prescription medications. Her examination was unremarkable except for a small right breast lump.

Initially, patient LJ had a difficult course on her nutritional protocol. Her apparent liver pain at times was severe enough to require MS Contin for a period of many months. She suffered episodes of fatigue and malaise for a period of six months, before gradually improving. When I saw her for a return evaluation on May 13, 1991 —a year after she had begun her nutritional protocol—she was feeling much stronger and her abdominal pains had largely resolved. Unfortunately, she began to feel so well that without my knowledge, she subsequently discontinued her protocol, assuming she was "cured." In early July 1991, she called me very distraught, having just suffered a grand mal seizure. At that time, she admitted she had been off her protocol for several months. A CT scan on July 11, 1991 revealed a high-density epidural mass of 2 mm on the left sphenoidal ridge and a small low density area (0.8 mm) in the right temporoparietal region. Both areas heterogeneously enhanced with contrast medium and were felt to be metastatic brain lesions.

After a lecture from me, patient LJ immediately resumed her full program, with rapid improvement in all symptoms. CT scans of both the head and abdomen on April 17, 1992 were completely normal. Her liver and brain tumors had completely regressed.

When last seen in May 1993, she was doing well and remained compliant with her nutritional regimen. She reported being in excellent health, with no complaints.

At this time, patient LJ has completed more than three years on her protocol, and is completely free of her once "terminal" disease.

Dr. Gonzalez presented these 25 cancer case studies to the NCI in 1993 and then updated the patient status information in 2001. Below are Dr. Gonzalez's personal notes with updated survival information:

Metastatic breast cancer. Does a modified program. Alive and well 10 years out now. This patient's survival status was updated again in 2016. Please refer to page 257 for this additional information.

ST. LUKE'S HOSPITAL

DENVER

PATHOLOGICAL LABORATORY

M __L. ⸱⸱⸱ J ⸱ 44 (⸱ ⸱ ⸱__   Case No. 00⸱ ⸱

Date: **10-30-** ⸱ D/T

Dr. Jennings   Room: **AMB**

PROVISIONAL DIAGNOSIS: **Mass, L. breast**

SPECIMEN: **A. Needle directed L. breast biopsy**
                           B. L. breast biopsy

GROSS DESCRIPTION:

A. The specimen consists of an irregular roughly spherical mass of predominantly adipose mammary tissue, averaging 4.4 cm. diam. Extending radially from it at one point is a thin silver-colored wire which extends 2.8 cm. into the mass. Surrounding the needle is an approximately 1.5 cm. ill-defined focus of soft tissue hemorrhage, most appearing fresh but several areas having a grey-tan appearance. This focus is in turn within glistening white gritty fibrous tissue that has multiple tiny foci of yellow-white spherical firm opacities.

B. The specimen consists of a portion of dense mammary adipose tissue, 4.3 x 2.2 x 1.1 cm., having at one pole a pink-tan slightly lobulated point of induration with ill-defined margins, approximately 0.7 cm. diameter. Sectioning reveals no stellate formation, gritty sensation on cutting, or chalk-streaking. There are some similar tiny blue-dome cysts, no cyst exceeding 0.2 cm. diameter. Parallel sectioning throughout reveals the described rubbery fibrous tissue admixed with adipose tissue, no gross signs suspicious of malignancy. CPR

MICROSCOPIC:

Microscopic examination of the first specimen demonstrate a malignant tumor in situ consisting of nests and cords of cells frequently with central lumens and a cribriform pattern (histologic grade 1). The cells making up the tumor demonstrate abundant poorly defined granular cytoplasm and relatively uniform, slightly enlarged and irregular nuclei with small nucleoli (cytologic grade 2).

DIAGNOSIS:

A. Biopsy of left breast: ductal carcinoma in situ.
B. Biopsy of left breast: Fibro-cystic mastopathy with atypical proliferation.

C. Philip Reynolds, M.D.

ST. LUKE'S HOSPITAL
DENVER
PATHOLOGICAL LABORATORY

Patient: L   , J   47   Case No. 00

Dr. Jennings   Date: 7-24-

PROVISIONAL DIAGNOSIS:

SPECIMEN:

Metastatic mammary carcinoma

Needle aspiration of liver

GROSS DESCRIPTION:

Received in formalin labeled with the patient's name is a single needle biopsy fragment of soft tan tissue measuring approximately 1.0 cm. in length and 0.1 in greatest diameter. Submitted in toto in a single cassette.

MICROSCOPIC:

Multiple sections, stained by H+E, reveal abnormal lobular architecture and evidence of portal fibrosis. The hepatocytes are characterized by variable sized nuclei, occasional prominent nucleoli and abundant cytoplasm with fatty degeneration and focal pigmentation. There are numerous atypical cells consistent with mammary carcinoma.

DIAGNOSIS:

Metastatic mammary carcinoma

C. Philip Reynolds, M. D.
Associate Pathologist
7-24-89

Patient Name ___L_____ , J____

History Number _99 92 94_____

Date of Visit _3/01/90_____

STANFORD UNIVERSITY HOSPITAL
STANFORD UNIVERSITY MEDICAL CENTER
STANFORD, CALIFORNIA 94305
DEPARTMENT OF MEDICINE
ONCOLOGY DAY CARE CENTER
Page 1   (415) 723-7621

Kyle Fink, M.D.
2005 Franklin
Denver, Colorado 80205

cc R. Lee Jennings, M.D.
    2005 Franklin
    Denver, Colorado 80205

Dear Dr. Fink:

We had the pleasure of seeing your patient, J   I   in Stanford Oncology Day Care Center today. Although her history is familiar to you, we will review it now for our records.

IDENTIFICATION AND CHIEF COMPLAINT: Patient is a 47-year old white female nine months S/P right lumpdectomy for infiltrating ductal carcinoma. She has known metastasis to the liver, and is here for a second opinion regarding adjuvant therapies.

HISTORY OF PRESENT ILLNESS: The patient is a woman who in October 1986 had a mammogram which showed a mass in the mid to upper outer quadrant of her left breast. She was lactating at the time and was seen by a surgeon who performed a biopsy. The diagnosis was ductal carcinoma in situ. No radiation was recommended, but the patient did stop nursing following the surgery as was suggested by her gynocologist. In July 1989 the patient was seen for a regular follow-up exam by Dr. Jennings who noted a mass in the lower outer quadrant of her right breast which was not detectable by mammogram. A lumpdectomy was performed after the biopsy showed infiltrating ductal carcinoma, poorly differentiated. No nodal dissection was performed at the patient's request. The tumor measured approximately 3 cm in diameter and the margin of the tumor was thought to be 2 mm from the deep margin of the the lumpdectomy specimen. At the time of surgery the patient's CEA was 195. A CT scan was done on 7/19/89 showing an increased area of density in the lateral right lobe of the liver. A needle biopsy performed 7/24/89 confirmed a metastasis. Estrogen receptor and progesterone receptor status of the tumor were negative. The DNA flow-cytometric measurement was classified as medium aneuploid. She was staged at III-B with T3NukM1. Workup and preparation for the lumpdectomy included bone scan on 7/13/89 which showed increased uptake in the region of C5 thought to be secondary to degenerative disease of the cervical spine in addition to increased uptake in the left supraorbital ridge. Plain films of the spine and cranial vault were obtained and thought to be within normal limits. Chest x-ray was also normal at this time. A complete blood count and general survey panel were all within normal limits with the exception of GGT at 38 and bilirubin at 1.7. This workup was completed at St. Lukes Hospital in Denver. Patient began a course of systemic CAF

15-317 (Rev. 3/86)

Patient Name _____ Le___ J_____

History Number ___ 99 92 94 _____

Date of Visit ___ 3/01/90 _____

STANFORD UNIVERSITY HOSPITAL
STANFORD UNIVERSITY MEDICAL CENTER
STANFORD, CALIFORNIA 94305
DEPARTMENT OF MEDICINE
ONCOLOGY DAY CARE CENTER
Page 2   (415) 723-7621

chemotherapy in August 1989 with weekly fractionated doses. Her response was good, but the patient developed early symtoms of adriamycin cardiomypathy detected by serial radionuclide angiography in November after 249 mg/m2 adriamyacin and declined further chemotherapy. Her CEA at 11/22/89 was 18.8. Since December 1989 patient has not been followed, but has been taking a vegetable immune stimulant called Thuja with some cooperation from a local surgeon in the Boulder area. Her family is anxious for her to explore other treatment options.

The patient has a history of breast cancer in both maternal and paternal grandmothers and aunts. She has two children ages 26 and 6. She has had five total pregnancies with one abortion and two miscarrages in addition to the living children. Age of first pregnancy was 21; menarche was at age 12. She is currently having regular menstrual cycles and had her last menstrual period on 2/26/90 which she thought was normal. She gives a history of use of birth control pills for approximately four years in 1965 and has never used DES. At present, her only complaints are of episodic nausea and some dyspnea with heavy exertion. She specifically denies decreased appetite, weight loss or bone pain.

PAST MEDICAL HISTORY: Remarkable for a motor vehicle accident at age 24 followed by a concussion. The patient believes the area of injury during her accicent may correspond with the left supraorbital ridge which is eliminated on the bone scan. Past surgery: appendectomy and removal of right ovarian cyst in 1956, S/P one abortion and tubal ligation in 1972. Microsurgery to reverse tubal ligation in 1982. Miscarriage in November 1982, followed by a pregnancy in 1983, carried to term, C-section. Cholecystectomy in January 1989. She is currently taking no medications except the Thuja extract. Patient has known drug allergy to ampicillian, and denies any history of nicotine or ethanol usage. She does admit to a distant history of marijuana smoking on an irregular basis. She denies any I.V. drug abuse.

FAMILY HISTORY: Remarkable for a mother who died at age 63 of heart failure. Father is currently living at age 78. He suffers from peripheral vascular disease and coronary disease. The patient has no siblings. The patient's children ages 25 and 5 are alive and well.

SOCIAL HISTORY: The patient is self-employed as a management consultant in Boulder, Colorado. She lives there with her husband, and her youngest child.

REVIEW OF SYSTEMS; Remarkable for asthma from animal danders which responds to ventolin inhalent. The remainder of the review of systems is not contributory.

15-317 (Rev. 3/86)

Patient Name ___L ⸱⸱⸱ , J___	**STANFORD UNIVERSITY HOSPITAL** STANFORD UNIVERSITY MEDICAL CENTER STANFORD, CALIFORNIA 94305
History Number ___99 92 94___	DEPARTMENT OF MEDICINE ONCOLOGY DAY CARE CENTER
Date of Visit ___3/01/90___	Page 3 (415) 723-7621

PHYSICAL EXAM: Reveals a moderately obese woman in no acute distress. Wt 60.4 kg, ht 157 cm, BP 110/70, P 80, temp 36.6.

Skin:
There are six or seven 3 or 4 cm lesions on the lower back which patient reports as having being biopsied two years earlier as pseudopsoriasis. There is a 1 cm nevus on the left anterior shoulder with irregular pigmentation, but a smooth margin.

HEENT:
Within normal limits.

Neck:
Supple without thyromegaly.

Nodes:
There is no palpable peripheral adenopathy.

Breasts:
Both breasts give evidence of mammary dysplasia. There are no visible lesions or skin changes. Both nipples are everted. Biopsy and lumpdectomy incisions show no erythema, exudate or drainage.

Chest:
Clear to auscultation and percussion.

Cardiac:
Regular rate and rhythm without murmurs, rubs or gallops. PMI cannot be appreciated.

Abdomen:
Obese and tender; some ascites. Positive bowel sounds. There is minor hepatosplenomegaly.

GU:
Deferred.

Extremities:
There is slight edema in the right medial upper arm. The remaining extremities are without clubbing, cyanosis or edema.

Neurologic:
Within normal limits.

LAB:
WBC 5300 with a differential of 63 polys, 27 lymphs, 10 monocytes; hgb 12.0; hct 33.4; platelets 202,000. General survey panel from today shows calcium 8.2 albumin 3.4, and GGT 34. CEA was 21.

X-RAYS:
Patient had x-ray studies of spine and chest today which were within normal limits. She hand carried both her initial and her most recent CTs (dated 7/19/89 and 11/22/89 and bone scan dated 7/13/89. We concur with the readings of these examinations which were performed at St. Lukes in Denver.

15-317 (Rev. 3/86)

Patient Name L___, J___

History Number 99 92 94

Date of Visit 3/01/90

STANFORD UNIVERSITY HOSPITAL
STANFORD UNIVERSITY MEDICAL CENTER
STANFORD, CALIFORNIA 94305
DEPARTMENT OF MEDICINE
ONCOLOGY DAY CARE CENTER
Page 4   (415) 723-7621

IMPRESSION: This is a 47-year-old woman S/P lumpdectomy for infiltrating ductal carcinoma of the right breast with metastasis to the lateral right lobe of the liver. The diagnosis is confirmed and the liver involvement has been documented by the Stanford Pathology Laboratory.

PLAN: We recommend the patient resume systemic therapy to include CMF chemotheraphy according to the Bonadonna protocol, i.e. Cytoxan 100mg/M2 p.o. each day on days 1-14, Methotrexate 40 mg/m2 I.V. days 1 and 8, and 5-FU 600 mg/m2 I.V. days 1 and 8. This cycle is repeated every 28 days as long as there is a control response with dosage reduction for leukopenia or throbocytopenia for each cycle. We recommend that this chemotherapy regimen be started as soon as possible.

Thank you for referring this patient to us. If we can be of any further assistance, please do not hesitate to call.

Sincerely,

Thomas M. Schieble   Frank E. Stockdale, M.D.
Medical Student   Professor of Medicine

nl, 3/2

15-317 (Rev. 3/86)

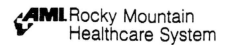 Rocky Mountain
Healthcare System

ST. LUKE'S HOSPITAL
DEPARTMENT OF RADIOLOGY

NUCLEAR MEDICINE BONE SCAN WHOLE BODY

The patient is a 47 year old woman with a history of breast cancer.
There are no prior bone scans.

Following intravenous injection of 21.9 millicurie of Technetium
labeled MDP scanning was performed over the entire skeleton.
Anterior and posterior whole body images and 8 camera views are
provided.

FINDINGS:

The distribution of activity in the soft tissues is normal. In the
bones there is noted a focus of uptake at the skull base near the
expected location of the anterior clinoids. There is increased
uptake seen in the supraorbital ridge and cervical spine, at C5, C4
and C3. Both right and left sides of the bone in C5 are noted to
be involved.

FINAL IMPRESSION:

There are multiple focal areas of increased activity in the spine
consistent with metastatic carcinoma.

        T. R. MUELLER, M.D.
        TRM: mmTo 7/13/89 09:56
        100

NAME:	L. , J	DATE:	7/13/89
ROOM:	BREAST	PHYS:	JENNINGS
ADM:		PHYS:	
HIST#:	0C	PHYS:	
XRAY#:		AGE:	47
SEX:	F		

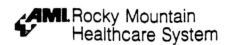**Rocky Mountain
Healthcare System**

ST. LUKE'S HOSPITAL
DEPARTMENT OF RADIOLOGY

HIGH-RESOLUTION SONOGRAM, ABDOMEN

Sector scans show normal size liver, with two hyperechoic masses in
the liver, the largest of these measured about 20 to 22 mm in the
lateral subcapsular portion of the right hepatic lobe superiorly.
A second, similar-shaped, hyperechoic nodule of about 10 mm is
present more inferiorly in the right hepatic lobe. Metastases
cannot be excluded and nuclear blood pool scan of the liver is
suggested. Head and body of the pancreas appear normal. No
hydronephrosis is seen at either kidney. No ascites is seen.

IMPRESSION:

Two hyperechoic hepatic masses, appearance suggests possible
cavernous hemangiomata, but metastasis isn't excluded. Further
evaluation with a nuclear labeled blood pool scan is suggested.

T.R. Mueller, M.D>
TRM:mmTo 7/18/89 09:55
100

NAME:	L J	DATE:	7/12/89
ROOM:	BREAST	PHYS:	JENNINGS
ADM#:		PHYS:	
HIST#:	OC	PHYS:	
XRAY#:		AGE:	47
SEX:	F		

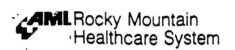**AML** Rocky Mountain Healthcare System

•

X-RAY JACKET

Corrected copy: This procedure was performed on 7-11-91. Dr. Steven Johnson noted error on original report.

SAINT LUKE'S HOSPITAL - DEPARTMENT OF RADIOLOGY

L.   J

7-11-91: CT SCAN BRAIN

Patient is a 49 year old woman with a history of breast cancer and known liver and bone metastases. She has recent slight left hemiparesis and vision disturbance.

Following oral contrast administration, serial axial 10 mm sections were performed of the brain prior to intravenous contrast. After intravenous injection of 150 cc's of Omnipaque scans were performed at 5 mm intravals.

IMPRESSION:

There is a high-density epidural mass of approximately 2 mm on the left sphenoidal ridge and a small low density area (approximately 0.8 mm) in the right temporoparietal region. Both areas were heterogeneously enhanced with contrast medium and appear to be metastatic brain lesions.

J.E. List, M.D.
D: 7/11/91 Time: 1330
T: 7/11/91 Time: 16:10
Tape #: 817
ID: JJG-V07D

L.   J
HIST #:   00
D.O.B.:
M.D.: Jennings
X-RAY #:

BOULDER COMMUNITY HOSPITAL
0 BALSAM, BOULDER, CO
-2179 (REPORTS)
PARTMENT OF IMAGING

MAPLETON CENTER FOR REHABILITATION
311 MAPLETON, BOULDER, CO
441-0473 (REPORTS)
DEPARTMENT OF IMAGING

X-RAY NO.

DATE PROCEDURE COMPLETED
04/17/92

-RAY FILE

IMAGING INTERPRETATION AND CONSULTATION

WHOLE BODY BONE SCAN

REASON FOR EXAMINATION: History of breast carcinoma and known liver metastases.

TECHNIQUE: 23.8mCi of 99m technetium-MDP were injected intravenously. Delayed images of the skeleton were obtained in anterior and posterior projections. There is no previous examination for comparison.

FINDINGS: There is very mild uptake in the region of a left facet joint at approximately C5. Though this may represent metastatic disease, I would think it would be more likely to represent very mild cervical spondylosis. The patient has a very mild scoliosis of the thoracic spine. Minimal increased uptake is seen in the right side of the mandible, probably secondary to dental disease.

IMPRESSION:

1. Focal very mild area of increased activity in the left side of the cervical spine, probably degenerative change

Stephen M. Miller, M.D./vgt

RADIOLOGISTS - K.F. DUBACH, M.D.   W.B. SEALE, M.D.   D.A. OPPENHEIMER, M.D.   P.D. KING, M.D.
K.D. MOORHEAD, M.D.   S.E. RECTOR, M.D.   C.R. BOWLES, M.D.   S.M. MILLER, M.D.

Q

L   J

BONE SCAN WHOLE BODY

PROBLEM: BREAST CA

LUCE,W.D.,M.D. / 900
cc: / 0

HOSP # :

F   49 DOB: 42
    CO   80302 (303) 449-3263
EXAM DATE: 04/17/92   EXAM TIME: 09:13
REPORT DATE: 04/17/92

PAT SS#:

GUAR: ROBERT S.
                ST

INS# 430   REL:
INSR

HUA001937556 3165 FRM-1

BOULDER COMMUNITY HOSPITAL   MAPLETON CENTER FOR REHABILITATION   X-RAY NO:

00 BALSAM, BOULDER, CO   311 MAPLETON, BOULDER, CO

)-2179 (REPORTS)   441-0473 (REPORTS)

DEPARTMENT OF IMAGING   DEPARTMENT OF IMAGING

DATE PROCEDURE COMPLETED: 04/17/92

X-RAY FILE   IMAGING INTERPRETATION AND CONSULTATION

CT SCAN/HEAD

REASON FOR EXAMINATION: History of metastatic breast carcinoma. Met in sphenoid ridge.

TECHNIQUE: Using the GE 9800 scanner, serial axial 10mm sections were performed through the brain prior to intravenous contrast. Subsequent scans were performed at 5mm intervals through the posterior fossa and 10mm intervals through the remainder of the brain after the intravenous administration of 150cc's of Omnipaque-300. Windowing was obtained for brain, blood and soft tissue.

FINDINGS: There is no mass or mass effect. There is a cavum septum pellucidum. There is no evidence of metastatic disease. The osseous structures are normal. The paranasal sinuses are normal.

IMPRESSION:

1. Normal CT scan of the head.

Stephen M. Miller, M.D./vgt

_____, M.D.

RADIOLOGISTS · K.P. DUBACH, M.D.   W.B. SEALE, M.D.   D.A. OPPENHEIMER, M.D.   P.D. KING, M.D.
K.D. MOORHEAD, M.D.   S.E. RECTOR, M.D.   C.R. BOWLES, M.D.   S.M. MILLER, M.D.

O

L.   J   HOSP # :
                                       F   49 DOB: 42
                             BOULDER, CO   80302 (303) 449-3263
CT HEAD WITH-WITHOUT CONTRAST   EXAM DATE: 04/17/92   EXAM TIME: 09:15
                             REPORT DATE: 04/17/92

PROBLEM: BREAST CA

                             PAT SS#:

LUCE,W.D.,M.D. / 900
cc: / 0

                             GUAR: ROBERT S.

                                   , CO   80302
                             INS# 430   REL:
                             INSR

HBA001937556 3169 FRM-3

4. Patient: LG
DOB 11/12/35

Patient LG is a 55 year-old white female with a history of metastatic breast cancer. She had been in good health when in mid-1984, she first noticed a right breast mass. After consulting her gynecologist, patient LG was referred to a surgeon for a breast biopsy, which was read as benign. However, within a month of the procedure, her health began to decline rapidly: she developed gradually worsening fatigue, paresthesias and chronic wheezing. Her internist reassured her, telling her "not to worry."

During early 1985, patient LG suffered a gradual weight loss, and then in April, 1985, her right breast and axillary region suddenly enlarged and became inflamed. Her physician thought she had an infected breast and prescribed antibiotics, but the breast swelling only worsened. Finally, in August 1985 she was admitted to Cabrini Medical Center in New York for evaluation. On exam, patient LG was found to have an 8 by 8 cm. mass, exhibiting inflammatory effect, and biopsy at that time confirmed infiltrating carcinoma. Hormone receptors were negative.

The tumor was thought far too large for resection, so a course of radiation was recommended. In September, 1985, patient LG began radiotherapy to the chest wall, eventually receiving six weeks of treatment for a total of 5100 rads. Then on November 11, 1985 at Cabrini, she underwent a right modified radical mastectomy. The pathology report describes carcinoma in 17/17 axillary nodes at all levels.

Shortly after surgery, patient LG began chemotherapy with CMF, a protocol she continued for two complete years. However, in August 1987, while still on therapy, she developed pain in her ribs and sternum. A bone scan September 1, 1987 documented increased activity in the sternum and two right anterior ribs. X-rays confirmed probable sternum metastases, but the rib lesions were thought more consistent with arthritis.

Because of her recurrence after prolonged aggressive chemotherapy, patient LG began investigating alternative approaches to cancer. She learned of my work and first came to my office on December 3, 1987, while she was still continuing chemotherapy. At that time, she complained of fatigue and severe depression, particularly worse after each dose of chemo. Physical exam was unrevealing.

In December 1987, patient LG began her nutritional protocol. She enjoyed rapid resolution of her bone pain and depression, as well as improvement in her overall health. Today, after 5.5 years, she still follows her nutritional regimen and is in excellent health. Periodically, she has received additional doses of single agent chemotherapy, usually methotrexate, from her oncologist.

Patient LG has not undergone repeat bone scans since the fall of 1987 so I cannot document regression of disease. Nonetheless, in the context of her 17/17 positive nodes, her large inflammatory primary tumor, and the occurrence of metastatic disease after two years on chemo, I believe her 5.5 years of healthy survival on her nutritional protocol makes her an unusual patient.

Dr. Gonzalez presented these 25 cancer case studies to the NCI in 1993 and then updated the patient status information in 2001. Below are Dr. Gonzalez's personal notes with updated survival information:

Metastatic breast cancer. Alive and well. No signs of disease 13 years out. This patient's survival status was updated again in 2016. Please refer to page 257 for this additional information.

Name   L. ... G. ...   Age **49** Sex **F**   Surg Path No   S85-

                                                            1216

Address   Location   Chart No

Date Spec. Rec'd   8-13-85   Date of Report   8-14-85   Service   Dr. Cammarat../Boyad

Clinical:

Nature of Specimen:

   Right Breast Mass (Frozen Section)

Pathological Description:
   GROSS (8-13-85): The specimen consists of a portion of breast tissue
   that measures 5.0 x 4.0 x 4.0 cm. An ill-defined area of 2.5 x 3.0 cm.
   formed by a firm, gritty tissue is noted 0.5 cm. from the nearest resected margin. Representative sections taken. Tissue submitted for
   ERA/PRA. Frozen Section Diagnosis: Duct Cell Carcinoma, Moderately
   Well Differentiated Infiltrating.

                                                            MTS/jg

   DIAGNOSIS: T04000-M81403 Duct Cell Carcinoma, Moderately Well
                               Differentiated Infiltrating, Intraductal

   NOTE: Tumor is seen inside lymphatic channels. A moderate lymphocytic
           infiltrate is noted.

   Respectfully submitted.

   M.T. Sabatini, M.D.

CHC 0266 5M REV 10/83
H-H, 78174

227 East 19th Street
New York, N.Y. 10003

SURGICAL PATHOLOGY REPORT

SURGICAL PATH. #: S85-

NAME: L   G   AGE: 49   SEX: F
ADDRESS:
ROOM: 1428   CHART#:
RECEIVED: 11-11-85   REPORTED: 11-12-85
SERVICE: Dr. Cammarata

CLINICAL:

NATURE OF SPECIMEN:
Right breast

PATHOLOGICAL DESCRIPTION:
GROSS (11-11-85): The specimen consists of a modified
radical mastectomy formed by an ellipse of skin containing
areola and nipple, subcutaneous tissue and underlying breast
tissue and axillary lymph nodes. The specimen measures 30.0
x 20.0 x 17.0 cm. in greatest dimensions. A recent surgical
scar of 6.0 cm. in length is noted around the areola. The
areola and nipple are not remarkable. The underlying tissue
contains extensive areas of induration and blue cyst
averaging 0.2 cm. in diameter. No residual tumor is noted.
The lymph nodes range in sizes from 0.5 upto 1.0 cm. in
diameter. Some of them appear firm. Representative sections
and lymph nodes submitted according to levels.
                         MTS/ie

DIAGNOSIS: T04000-M32100   Right Modified Radical Mastectomy
                           with No Residual Tumor
                           Balance of Breast with Duct
            T04000-M33400   Ectasia, Cysts and
            T04000-M49000   Stromal Fibrosis
            T08000-M80103* Three out of Three Lymph Nodes,
                           Upper Group, with Secondary
                           Carcinoma
            T08000-M80103* Seven out of Seven Lymph Nodes,
                           Middle Group, with Secondary
                           Carcinoma
            T08000-M80103   Seven out of Seven Lymph Nodes,
                           Lower Group, with Secondary
                           Carcinoma

Respectfully submitted.

M.T. Sabatini, M.D.

GRAMERCY RADIOLOGY GROUP, P.C.

201 EAST 19th STREET

NEW YORK, N.Y. 10003

(212) 460-8100

DANIELE SALVIONI, M.D.
GUIDO PADULA, M.D.
CHERYL BYK, M.D.
AMADO DOLORICO, M.D.
ALAN BERNSTEIN, M.D.

Sept. 1, 1987

Mirjana, Valancic, M.D.
70 E. 10 St.
New York, N.Y. 10003   RE: L   G

BONE SCAN: 9/1/87

Ninety minutes after the intravenous administration of 20 millicuries
of Tc99m MDP, multiple films of the axial skeleton were obtained on
the gamma camera.

There is diffuse increased activity of the radiopharmaceutical noted
in the entire spine and the large joints of the body as well as the
first metatarsal phalangeal joints bilaterally all compatible with
arthritis. There is some focal uptake of the radiopharmaceutical
in the mid aspect of the sternum and if clinically warranted,
suggest x-ray of the sternum for further evaluation. There is also
some slight increased activity noted in two right anterior ribs and
a right rib series is recommended for further evaluation.

Renal excretion is symmetrical.

IMPRESSION: ABNORMAL FOCI OF INCREASED ACTIVITY STERNUM AND
                   TWO RIGHT ANTERIOR RIBS. RECOMMEND X-RAYS.

                   ARTHRITIS.

Thank you for referring this patient.

                                         Very truly yours,

                                         Cheryl Byk M.D.

                                         Cheryl Byk,M.D.

CB/ss

GRAMERCY RADIOLOGY GROUP, P.C.
201 EAST 19th STREET
NEW YORK, N. Y. 10003

(212) 660-5300

DANIELE SALIVONE, M.D.
GUIDO PADULA, M.D.
CHERYL BYK, M.D.
AMADO DOLORICO, M.D.
ALAN BERNSTEIN, M.D.

September 9, 1987

Angelo Cammarata, M.D.
55 East 87 Street
New York, New York 10028   RE: L.   , G

BILATERAL RIBS AND STERNUM - 9/9/87

STERNUM:
Oblique and lateral projections of the sternum reveal marked
irregularity to the cortex of the proximal body of the sternum.
In addition, distally, there is some periosteal reaction in
the body of the sternum and these findings when correlating
with the abnormal Bone Scan of 9/1/87 most likely represents
sternal metastasis. Suggest clinical correlation.

BILATERAL RIBS:
PA and oblique projections of the right ribs reveal no evidence
for a fracture. In addition, there was no evidence for an
osteolytic or osteoblastic metastasis.   There is no abnormality
on the left.

Thank you for referring this patient.

Yours truly,

Cheryl Byk, M.D.

CB:cb

5. Patient: SH
DOB: 4/18/39

Patient SH is a 54 year-old white female rancher from Colorado with a history of metastatic breast cancer. As a teenager, she received radiation to the chest for treatment of keloids but otherwise was in good health until late 1986, when she developed a left breast mass. Subsequently, on January 8, 1987 at Lovelace Medical Center, Albuquerque, patient SH underwent a modified radical mastectomy. The pathology report documents adenocarcinoma, with metastatic disease in 8/23 nodes. There was no evidence of distant metastases on chest X-ray, bone scan or abdominal ultrasound. Post surgery, patient SH completed a six-month course of chemotherapy with CMF, followed by tamoxifen.

Patient SH did well until late 1990 when she developed chronic pleuritic chest pain. A chest X-ray on April 16, 1991, revealed a left pleural effusion that was then aspirated on April 18, 1991: cytologic examination was positive for malignant cells. A bone scan on May 8, 1991 was negative. In April, tamoxifen was discontinued and patient SH began Megace, but her symptoms only worsened. A repeat chest X-ray on August 28, 1991 demonstrated a persistent pleural effusion. Aggressive chemotherapy was suggested, but refused by the patient, who at that point was already investigating alternative cancer approaches.

Patient SH learned of my work and first came to my office on September 12, 1991. At that time, she reported severe DOE and cough. She was taking Megace 80 mg BID. Her examination was notable for bilateral breast implants and decreased breath sounds on the left.

She discontinued Megace and began her nutritional protocol after returning to Colorado in September 1991. Within weeks, she reported a significant improvement in her breathing and well being, and since that time she has remained very compliant with her program. When last seen on April 1, 1993, she reported feeling "wonderful," better than she had in years. Her respiratory symptoms had long resolved and her pulmonary examination was normal. A repeat chest X-ray April 30, 1993 showed no evidence of pleural effusion or mass lesion. Patient SH has now completed nearly two years on her nutritional regimen and appears to be disease free.

Dr. Gonzalez presented these 25 cancer case studies to the NCI in 1993 and then updated the patient status information in 2001. Below are Dr. Gonzalez's personal notes with updated survival information:

Widely metastatic breast cancer. Died April 1998 after 6.5 years.

LOVELACE MEDICAL CENTER, INC. • 5400 GIBSON BLVD. S.E. • ALBUQUERQUE, NEW MEXICO 87108

SPECIMEN: Right breast tissue

HISTORY:

LOVELACE CLINIC
PATHOLOGY DEPT.

GROSS:

One container labeled with name and number. There is an irregular fragment of breast tissue measuring 3.7 x 2.4 x .9 cm. It appears to consist of about 25% parenchyma and the remainder fat. External and cut surfaces are grossly unremarkable. The specimen is sectioned in its short axis and all submitted in three cassettes. RF:mb

MICROSCOPIC:

Several portions of this specimen demonstrate an infiltrating epithelial neoplasm. In most fields, the neoplastic cells have the appearance of lobular carcinoma, with formation of solid clusters of cells, or a single-file pattern of infiltration. Cytologically the cells have dark and uniform round to oval nuclei, and moderate to large amounts of clear or faintly amphophilic cytoplasm of polygonal shape. In some foci, small ductular structures are formed by the neoplastic elements. Foci of possible lymphatic permeation are identified, but this cannot be differentiated with certainty from retraction artifact.

DIAGNOSIS:

RIGHT BREAST TISSUE, INFILTRATING ADENOCARCINOMA, MIXED LOBULAR AND DUCTAL TYPE.

(9

RF:mb

R. FEDDERSON, M. D.
PATHOLOGY RESIDENT

SIGNATURE OF PATHOLOGIST

T.L. CHIFFELLE, M.D.   P. AVASTHI, M.D.
LEE GATES, III, M.D.   T.D. STUART, M.D.
PATHOLOGISTS

1-605 ℗

PATIENT NO.	,	CLINIC
NAME	S. , H.	
BIRTHDATE	39	
DOCTOR	THOMAS	
DATE	87	
	CHC: 1501: 4507	
PATH. NO.	S- -87	

PATHOLOGY REPORT

PAGE 1.

LOVELACE MEDICAL CENTER, INC. • 5400 GIBSON BLVD. S.E. • ALBUQUERQUE, NEW MEXICO 87108

SPECIMEN: 1. Left breast mass - tissue - frozen section
2. Breast tissue, Right   right 12 AM 25
Suspicious fullness - tail of Spence - U/I breast

HISTORY: invasive adenocarcinoma right breast

.VELACE CLINIC
.ATHOLOGY DEPT.

GROSS:

The specimen consists of 4 x 3 x 2 cm. somewhat fatty breast tissue fragment
which on sectioning reveals pale tan firm breast parenchyma without any
grossly identifiable infiltrating lesion. Also received is another
4 x 3 x 2 cm. fatty breast tissue in which a minimum area of breast parenchyma
is noticed. No grossly identifiable lesions are present. The specimen
is sectioned and all the breast tissue is totally embedded.
PA:mb

FROZEN SECTION DIAGNOSIS--

Left breast biopsy-Mild fibrocystic disease. P. Avasthi

The second specimen consists of fibrofatty breast which measures 24 x 18 x 5 cm.
in greatest dimension and is covered on one aspect by 24 x 8.5 cm. elliptical
skin fragment. The nipple and areola are identified and are grossly unremarkable.
3.5 cm. lateral to the nipple to the areolar margin there is a vertical
4.5 cm. recent surgical incision which is closed with sutures. The surrounding
skin has yellowish purplish blue discoloration. The deeper portion of the specimen
includes intact fascia with a few adherent skeletal muscle fibers. On sectioning
the breast is moderately fatty with some amount of tan, pink breast parenchyma
in it. No other lesions are grossly identified. The site of previous biopsy
is indicated by a cavitary defect full of blood. This is noticed 1 cm. deeper to
the skin and extends close to the deep margin of resection. The fibrous fascia
at the area of surgical defect is 0.1 cm. only. The cavitary is 3.5 x 3.5 cm.
in greatest dimension. No grossly identifiable tumor is present at the site of
biopsy. The outer lateral portion of the specimen includes 9 x 5 x 2 cm. of
fibrofatty tissue. The apex is indicated by black suture. Multiple hard lymph
nodes are palpable in this area. The largest lymph node measures 3.5 x 3 cm.
One of the lymph nodes noticed at the apex near the silk suture grossly appears
to be positive. The sections are embedded as follows: "A" from the distal most
site of dissection, lymph nodes; "B" from the middle group of lymph nodes; "C"
from the proximal group of lymph nodes; "D" from the breast tissue away from the
biopsy site; "T" from the biopsy site; "M" from the deep margin of resection at
the biopsy site; "N" from the nipple.

CONTINUED...

SIGNATURE OF PATHOLOGIST

T.L. CHIFFELLE, M.D.   P. AVASTHI, M.D.
LEE GATES, III, M.D.   T.D. STUART, M.D.
            PATHOLOGISTS
1-605 ℗

PATIENT NO.	
NAME	S ... H
BIRTHDATE	39
DOCTOR	Thomas
DATE	1 8 87
PATH. NO.	516, 1509- 1743
	S-. -87

PATHOLOGY REPORT

LOVELACE MEDICAL CENTER, INC. • 5400 GIBSON BLVD. S.E. • ALBUQUERQUE, NEW MEXICO 87108

SPECIMEN:

   Refer to Page 1. for description.   '97 JAN 12 AM 11.25

HISTORY:

                                          LOVELACE CLINIC
                                          PATHOLOGY DEPT.

      MICROSCOPIC:

      1. The sections reveal fibrofatty breast tissue showing scattered areas
      of cystic distension of the ducts or lobules with epithelial proliferation.
      Apocrine metaplasia is noticed. There is ductular epitheliosis but no
      distinctive cellular atypia.

      2. Sections from the previous site of biopsy reveal residual infiltrating
      small foci of adenocarcinoma which extends to the deep margin of resection.
      In addition, there is proliferation of fibriblasts and blood vessels with
      organizing inflammation.   Sections away from the previous biopsy site generally
      indicates fibrocystic disease. A small focus of adenocarcinoma this area, however,
      does show proliferation of the fibroblasts and probably in continuation with
      the previous biopsy site. The other sections show mild fibrocystic disease.
      The sections from the nipple are unremarkable. Sections from the large lymph
      nodes show partial or subtotal replacement by the metastatic garxi adenocarcinoma
      both duct and lobular type. The perinodal adipose tissue is not infiltrated
      by the tumor.

      DIAGNOSIS:

      LEFT BREAST BIOPSY, FIBROCYSTIC DISEASE.

      2. RIGHT BREAST: MODIFIED RADICAL MASTECTOMY, RESIDUAL MIXED LOBULAR AND
                         DUCTAL ADENOCARCINOMA, MODERATELY DIFFERENTIATED AT THE
                         PREVIOUS SITE OF BIOPSY WITH METASTATIC TUMOR IN
                         EIGHT OUT OF TWENTY-THREE LYMPH NODES INCLUDING THE MOST
                         DISTAL GROUP OF LYMPH NODES NEAR THE SUTURE.

                         FIBROCYSTIC DISEASE.

SIGNATURE OF PATHOLOGIST

T.L. CHIFFELLE, M.D.   P. AVASTHI, M.D.
LEE GATES, III, M.D.   T.D. STUART, M.D.

1-605 ℗   PATHOLOGISTS

PATIENT NO.	392
NAME	S. ... H.
BIRTHDATE	.. . 39
DOCTOR	Thomas
DATE	1 8 87
	1516,1509-1743
PATH. NO.	S-140-87

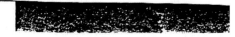

PATHOLOGY REPORT

LOVELACE, INC.

NAME: S.   H.   MRN: DOB: 18-Apr-39

REF. PHYSICIAN: MICHAEL L COYLE MD   WARD/UNIT: GENERAL SURGERY

ORDER #:492A-041791   ROOM#: OP   DATE OF EXAM: 17-Apr-91

CLINICAL DATA:
CHEST PA LAT F/U PLEURAL EFFUSION

Exam: XR CHEST 2 VIEW

PA AND LATERAL CHEST: 4-17-91.

IMPRESSION: THE MOST RECENT AVAILABLE COMPARISON IS DATED 7-20-88.
            THERE IS A RELATIVELY LARGE LEFT SIDED PLEURAL EFFUSION
            PRESENT. IT OBSCURES THE LEFT HEART MARGIN MAKING IT
            DIFFICULT TO ASSESS HEART SIZE. THERE IS A SMUDGY AREA OF
            DENSITY IMMEDIATELY ABOVE THIS PLEURAL EFFUSION ON THE PA
            VIEW AND THIS MAY REPRESENT SOME INFILTRATION PROBABLY
            PROJECTING POSTERIORLY ON THE LATERAL VIEW. UPPER PORTION
            OF LEFT LUNG IS CLEAR AND ALL THE RIGHT LUNG IS CLEAR.
            SHARP RIGHT LATERAL COSTOPHRENIC ANGLE. NO DEFINITE HILAR OR
            MEDIASTINAL MASSES. BONY THORAX APPEARS INTACT.

            DL   4-19-91
            T: 4-22-91

                    signed: RICHARD S. NENOFF, MD

RSN/ph

NAME: S   H   MRN:

TRANSCRIBED DATE: 22-Apr-91 TIME: 06:50   PRINTED:24-Apr-91

S .   , H.   7/29/91   Dr. Anderson

LMC#

PROBLEM LIST: Recurrent breast cancer.

Mrs. S   us states she is feeling well. She does not have her chest discomfort. She gets fatigued fairly quickly.

OBJECTIVE: On examination she has no palpable nodes. Breast sounds are diminished at least half the way up the left side of the chest. She has no obvious skin recurrence. No hepatomegaly. She has a distended vein in her left leg over the kneecap which flattens out when the patient becomes recumbent.

Chest x-ray was taken and reviewed. The patient has fluid almost 2/3 of the way up on the left side of the chest. This is slightly more than the last x-ray from the 20th of May.

ASSESSMENT: The patient has a significant amount of fluid which would make be think that the Megace is not working particularly well, although the patient has had good symptomatic relief and a CEA that went from 5.4 to 1.7.

PLAN: We will see what her CEA now. If it continues to be low, I guess that I would keep her on the Megace for awhile. If it bumps up, perhaps we should consider changing her therapy, maybe even tapping her again.

TA/sms   Thomas Anderson, M.D.
7/29/91 7/30/91   HEMATOLOGY/ONCOLOGY

PATIENT NAME: S... ...,H
        UNIT NO:

EXAMS: CHEST-PA + LATERAL
EXAM DATE: 04/30/93

Chest PA and lateral 04/30/93 compared with 04/16/91.

Lungs are slightly hyperinflated compatible with chronic obstructive
pulmonary disease. There has been a right mastectomy and there is an
inflatable implant present. No acute pulmonary infiltrates. Heart
size is normal.

        IMPRESSION: CHRONIC OBSTRUCTIVE PULMONARY DISEASE. RIGHT
        MASTECTOMY.

                        VAUGHN A. JOHNSON, M.D.

CC:

TRANSCRIBED DATE/TIME: 04/30/93 (1719)
TRANSCRIPTIONIST: PG
PRINTED DATE/TIME: 04/30/93 (1720)
PAGE 1

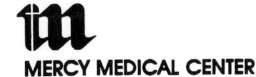

MERCY MEDICAL CENTER

375 E. Park Avenue • Durango, Colorado 81301 • 303/247-4311

NAME: S... ,H
PHYS: GONZALEZ,NICHOLAS J
DOB: 39   AGE: 54   SEX: F
ACCT NO: M000...   LOCATION: DI
STATUS: OUT
RADIOLOGY NO: 00...

6. Patient: SK
DOB: 6/4/49

Patient SK is a 44 year-old woman with a history of fibrocystic breast disease and breast cancer. She had been in good health when in the fall of 1990, she first noticed a breast mass. In October of 1990, biopsy of the breast mass revealed lobular carcinoma. Patient SK subsequently refused the recommended surgery, and instead went to Mexico for a trial of unorthodox therapy. Upon returning home to Pennsylvania, she agreed to surgery and on December 21, 1990 underwent partial mastectomy with axillary sampling at Reading Hospital Medical Center (Pennsylvania). The pathology report describes adenocarcinoma, with all sampled nodes negative for metastatic disease. However, the surgical margin was not clear microscopically. Subsequently, a bone scan in January of 1991 was clear, but a liver/spleen scan documented hepatic abnormalities. An MRI of the abdomen on January 7, 1991 demonstrated seven liver lesions, consistent with metastatic disease.

Patient SK then completed a one-month course of radiation consisting of 5000 rads to the chest wall. After she finished radiation in February 1991, liver biopsy and chemotherapy were suggested but adamantly refused.

Instead, patient SK decided to pursue my therapy and was first seen in my office on March 5, 1991. At that time, she had no complaints. She was taking tamoxifen 20 mg BID. Her examination was notable only for absent left breast with radiation dermatitis.

In October 1991, patient SK discontinued tamoxifen, preferring to rely solely on her nutritional regimen. At present, she has now completed more than two years on her protocol, remains a very compliant patient and is in excellent health. A follow-up MRI of the abdomen on November 23, 1992 revealed four lesions in the liver, two in the anterior segment measuring 1.5 and 2.0 cm.; a third lesion in the posterior segment of the right lobe and measuring 7.5 cm. The fourth lesion was described adjacent to the calciform ligament and measuring 2.0 cm. These are reported to be unchanged from the January 1991 study: however, an additional three hepatic lesions documented on the earlier report were not evident in the November 1992 scan. She appears to have enjoyed significant regression of her liver disease since beginning her nutritional program.

Dr. Gonzalez presented these 25 cancer case studies to the NCI in 1993 and then updated the patient status information in 2001. Below are Dr. Gonzalez's personal notes with updated survival information:

Metastatic breast cancer. Switched to a treatment in the Islands where she had an explosion while off her Gonzalez program. She died. Survived 5 years.

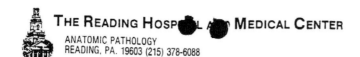

THE READING HOSPITAL AND MEDICAL CENTER

ANATOMIC PATHOLOGY
READING, PA. 19603 (215) 378-6088

I. Donald Stuard, M.D. - Director of Pathology

Patient: S. , K.	Patient Type: AMBULATORY
Med. Rec. No: (000010	Patient Loc/Room:
DOB/Sex: . 49 FEMALE	Admission Date: 11/12/90
Soc. Sec. No:	Specimen Received: 11/12/90 1301
Physician(s): WADEMAN, ROSS L	

SURGICAL PATHOLOGY

Surgery Date: 11/12/90   Accession: S-90-18757

SPECIMEN:

BX LEFT BREAST TISSUE

GROSS DESCRIPTION:

Received in formalin are two irregular fragments of fibrofatty tissue. The smaller fragment is firm to palpation, light tan in color, and measures 1.0 x 0.6 x 0.5 cm. The second fragment is larger measuring 2.5 x 1.5 x 1.0 cm. Frozen section diagnosis: infiltrating mammary carcinoma. Favor lobular carcinoma. A majority of the smaller specimen is frozen for hormone receptor assay. The remaining specimen is entirely submitted in three blocks. JHB/a

DIAGNOSIS:

BREAST, LEFT, BIOPSY:
--INFILTRATING LOBULAR CARCINOMA OF BREAST   8523
--ASSOCIATED MICROCALCIFICATIONS
--MARKED PERINEURAL INVASION

JHB/K
11/13/90 15:03

Jerry H. Broman, M.D.
Pathologist

End of Report   PATHOLOGY REPORT   Patient: S. , K.

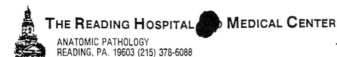

THE READING HOSPITAL MEDICAL CENTER
ANATOMIC PATHOLOGY
READING, PA. 19603 (215) 378-6088

I. Donald Stuard, M.D. - Director of Pathology

```
Patient: S     , K                      Patient Type:      AMBULATORY
Med. Rec. No: (0000)0                    Patient Loc/Room:
_OB/Sex:         49 FEMALE               Admission Date:    12/21/90
Soc. Sec. No:                            Specimen Received: 12/24/90  1610
Physician(s): WADEMAN, ROSS L
              PROBST, SUSAN J
              FAMILY MEDICAL CTR
```

SURGICAL PATHOLOGY

Surgery Date: 12/21/90   Accession: S-90-

SPECIMEN:
1) Portion left breast, 2) Left axillary contents

CLINICAL FINDINGS:
Adenocarcinoma left breast
Left partial mastectomy and axillary sampling

GROSS DESCRIPTION:
Specimens arrive in two containers fresh.

Container 1 is labeled "portion left breast". The specimen consists of a skin ellipse with underlying fatty breast tissue and skeletal muscle at the deep margin. It weighs 40 grams. The skin ellipse is 6.7 x 1.8 cm. Approximately in the mid portion of this there is a well healed surgical incision with still retains some sutures which is about 3 cm. in length. The underlying fatty breast tissue is up to 5.8 x 2 cm. The surgical margins are inked prior to further examination. No tumor is grossly visible at the external margins. Specimen is step sectioned at about 5 mm. intervals from the deep aspect towards the skin. Most of the parenchyma is occupied by a linear scar-like area which is about 3.5 x 1.2 cm. x 4 cm. This is unusually firm and some of the edges have glistening tan areas of suspicious for residual tumor. Tumor approaches grossly but does not definitely involve the margins. Multiple representative sections submitted following fixation.

Container 2 is labeled "left axillary contents". The specimen weighs 4 grams and consists of 4 to 5 cc's of yellow pink fatty tissue. This tissue is placed into Carnoy's fixative and any lymph nodes identified following fixation will be submitted. MLF/a

MICROSCOPIC DESCRIPTION:
Multiple sections show rather extensive residual tumor representing most or all of the scar like area noted grossly. Most of the tumor is infiltrating and grows in lobular fashion as "indian files" and "targetoid" fashion surrounding breast ducts. Focally, insitu tumor is seen filling and expanding breast ducts growing in a sheet like pattern in some areas and in a cribriform pattern in other ducts. Tumor cells are medium sized and have eosinophilic cytoplasm and enlarged nuclei with a granular chromatin pattern. There is perineural invasion as well as extension into skeletal muscle. In several areas, tumor approaches the inked margins and in at least one section (slide G) is seen at the inked surgical resection margin. There is no definite invasion of the attached skin. MLF/g

DIAGNOSIS:
1) PORTION LEFT BREAST:

Continued ...   PATHOLOGY REPORT   Patient: S

Proof of Concept

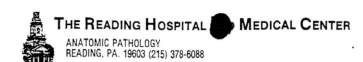

THE READING HOSPITAL MEDICAL CENTER

ANATOMIC PATHOLOGY
READING, PA. 19603 (215) 378-6088

I. Donald Stuard, M.D. - Director of Pathology

```
                              Patient Loc: ASG      Room:           Date: 12/26/9
                              Admitting Physician: WADEMAN, ROSS L
DEPARTMENT OF PATHOLOGY            Sex: FEMALE     Patient Name: S.    ,K.
THE READING HOSPITAL AND MEDICAL CENTER DOB:    ./49   Med. Rec. No:
```

SURGICAL PATHOLOGY

Surgery Date: 12/21/90   Accession: S-90-

DIAGNOSIS:

    --RECENT SURGICAL SITE WITH EXTENSIVE RESIDUAL INTRADUCTAL AND
      INFILTRATING CARCINOMA WITH DUCTAL AND LOBULAR FEATURES,
      TUMOR FOCALLY INVOLVES SURGICAL MARGINS (SEE MICROSCOPIC)   85003
    --FIBROCYSTIC CHANGES

    2) LEFT AXILLARY CONTENTS:
        --SIX LYMPH NODES, NO TUMOR IDENTIFIED (O/6)

    MLF/G
    12/26/90 12:05

                              Margaret L. Freeman, M.D.
                              Pathologist

End of Report   PATHOLOGY REPORT   Patient: S   ,K

54

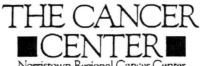

THE CANCER
■CENTER■
Norristown Regional Cancer Center
Division of Radiation Oncology

Brown & Powell Streets
Norristown, PA 19401
(215) 278-2510

February 20, 1991

Division of Radiation Oncology
Luther W. Brady, M.D., *Medical Director*
Jeffrey I. Damsker, M.D.
Scot A. Fisher, D.O.
William Serber, M.D.

Michael G. Stambaugh, M.S.
Radiological Physicist

K.   S
251 Faber Road
Reading, PA 19606

END TREATMENT NOTE

John Loughead, M.D.
223 East Lancaster Avenue
Shillington, PA 19607

Dear Dr. Loughead,

As you know, Mrs. S____ had excision of a small infiltrating
lobular carcinoma of the left breast on 11/12/90 and reexcision
with axillary dissection on 12/21. Six axillary nodes were
negative but residual tumor was present in the breast with
muscle invasion and microscopic tumor present at the surgical
resection margin. She has now completed a course of postoperative radiation treatment to the residual breast and
chest wall. The 6 MV beam was used (except for 5 treatments
with 18 MV when the 6 MV beam was inoperative) with tangential
fields and between 1/15 and 2/20/91 she received a tumor dose
of 5000 cGy. At present there is a moderate erythema which
is asymptomatic and should heal without difficulty.

She undoubtedly has extensive liver metastases, as noted on
scan and MRI. Tumor ER and PR were elevated and she is on
Tamoxifen. She will not consider chemotherapy. She says she
has no symptoms and after the first day or two she has been
quite cheerful.

I have asked her to return in 1 month for observation.

Very truly yours,

William Serber, M.D.

WS/smk
pc: Susan Probst, M.D.
     Luther Brady, M.D.
     Ross L. Wademan, M.D.

A cooperative venture by affiliates of Suburban General Corporation and Sacred Heart Health System.

Berks Imaging Center, Ltd.

1330 Penn Avenue, Wyomissing, Pennsylvania 19610   (215) 373-3100

DIAGNOSTIC X-RAY • MAMMOGRAPHY • ULTRASOUND

JONATHAN L. STOLZ, M.D.	LAURENCE A. CITRO, M.D.
MICHAEL E. GORDON, M.D.	LAWRENCE M. KAPLAN, M.D.

NAME: K   S   DATE: 01-0 -91   NO:

ADDRESS: , PA 19606

PHYSICIAN: ROSS WADEMAN, M.D.   BIRTHDATE: -49

MRI OF LIVER

IMPRESSION: MULTIPLE LESIONS SEEN ON HEAVY WEIGHTED T2 IMAGES. HEMANGIOMAS VERSUS METASTASIS; SUGGEST LIVER BLOOD POOL SCANNING; SEE COMMENT.

COMMENT: THE MRI OF THE LIVER WAS PERFORMED IN THE AXIAL PLANE WITH T1 AND MULTI-ECHO SEQUENCING AS WELL AS HEAVY WEIGHTED T2 SEQUENCES.

THE STUDY CONFIRMS THE PRESENCE OF MULTIPLE ABNORMALITIES SEEN ON THE T1-WEIGHTED WITH LOW SIGNAL INTENSITY WITH A LARGE LESION SEEN IN THE RIGHT LOBE OF THE LIVER AND MULTIPLE SMALLER LESIONS SEEN THROUGHOUT THE LIVER. A TOTAL OF APPROXIMATELY 7 LESIONS ARE SEEN.

ON THE T2 SEQUENCES INCREASED SIGNAL IS SEEN. ON THE HEAVILY WEIGHTED T2 SEQUENCE THE SIGNAL IS INCREASED SLIGHTLY MORE. IT INCREASES WITH THE RELATIONSHIP TO THE LIVER ITSELF.

THE DIFFERENTIAL DIAGNOSIS IS BETWEEN MULTIPLE HEMANGIOMAS AND METASTATIC DISEASE.

AT PRESENT NON-INVASIVE IMAGING STUDIES FALL SHORT IN ITS ABILITY TO MAKE A DEFINITIVE DIAGNOSIS BETWEEN THESE TWO LESIONS. HOWEVER, A HIGHER SPECIFICITY MAY BE OBTAINED BY UTILIZING BLOOD POOL TECHNETIUM SCANS WITH OR WITHOUT SPEC.

JONATHAN L. STOLZ, M.D.

LLC
DICT: 01/07/91
TRANS: 01/08/91

If the above Radiographic Report does not correlate with the clinical or pathological findings, please notify the office

Berks Imaging Center, Ltd.

1330 Penn Avenue, Wyomissing, Pennsylvania 19610   (215) 373-3100

DIAGNOSTIC X-RAY • MAMMOGRAPHY • ULTRASOUND • MRI

JONATHAN L. STOLZ, M.D.   MICHAEL E. GORDON, M.D.
LAURENCE A. CITRO, M.D.   LAWRENCE M. KAPLAN, M.D.   RICHARD A. HEIDEN, M.D.

NAME: K   S.   DATE: 11-23-92   NO:

ADDRESS: .   . READING, PA 19 .

PHYSICIAN: NICHOLAS GONZALEZ, M.D.   BIRTHDATE: -49
            737 PARK AVENUE
            NEW YORK, NY 10021

MRI OF ABDOMEN/LIVER:

IMPRESSION: NO CHANGE IN MULTIPLE LESIONS SEEN WITHIN THE
LIVER. FINDINGS CONSISTENT WITH HEMANGIOMA OR
INDULENT METS.

COMMENT: MRI OF THE LIVER WAS OBTAINED ACCORDING TO STANDARD
PROTOCOLS. PARTICULAR EMPHYSIS WAS PLACED ON THE HEAVILY T2-WEIGHTED
IMAGES.

CURRENTLY, FOUR LESIONS ARE IDENTIFIED. TWO LIE IN THE ANTERIOR
SEGMENT OF THE RIGHT LOBE AND MEASURE 1.5 AND 2.0 CM IN MAXIMUM
DIMENSION RESPECTIVELY. A THIRD LESION IS ALMOST AS LARGE AS THE
UNDERLYING KIDNEY AND LIES IN THE POSTERIOR SEGMENT OF THE RIGHT LOBE,
MEASURING AT LEAST 7.5 CM IN MAXIMUM DIMENSION. THE FOURTH LESION LIES
MORE INFERIORLY ADJACENT TO THE CALCIFORM LIGAMENT. THIS ALSO MEASURES
2.0 CM.

IMPORTANTLY, THERE HAS BEEN ABSOLUTELY NO CHANGE IN THE VOLUME OR
MORPHOLOGY OF THESE INTRAHEPATIC LESIONS SINCE THE PRIOR EXAMINATION OF
JANUARY 7, 1991. THEY HAVE THE IMAGING CHARACTERISTICS OF HEMANGIOMAS,
I.E.: LOW T1-WEIGHTED SIGNAL AND HIGH T2-WEIGHTED SIGNAL. OTHER
ENTITIES SUCH AS METASTASIS OR OTHER BENIGN LESIONS OF THE LIVER ARE
PROBABLY NOT RESPONSIBLE FOR THESE FINDINGS.

WE WOULD RECOMMEND CORRELATION WITH OTHER MODALITIES (DYNAMIC CT,
RADIONUCLIDE STUDY, ULTRASOUND, OR EVEN ANGIOGRAM) WHICH MAY HELP GIVE A
DEFINITIVE DIAGNOSIS OF HEMANGIOMA.

RICHARD A. HEIDEN, M.D.

LLG
DICT: 11/24/92
TRANS: 11/24/92

7. Patient: WC
DOB: 1/11/39

Patient WC is a 54 year-old white female with a history of breast cancer. She had previously been in good health when routine mammography in October of 1991 revealed a suspicious breast mass. Subsequently, on November 13, 1991, patient WC underwent biopsy and lumpectomy, with removal of a 2.1 cm. tumor. The pathology report describes in situ and infiltrating ductal carcinoma. No nodes were sampled: however, a bone scan on December 2, 1991 demonstrated increased uptake in the right proximal femur, and an MRI on January 6, 1992 confirmed a lesion on the right greater trochanter consistent with metastatic disease. Radiation and chemotherapy were proposed but refused by the patient.

Patient WC knew of my work and first came to my office on January 15, 1992. At that time, she reported fatigue and right hip pain, but otherwise had no complaints. She was taking Thyrolar II and SloBid. Her examination was notable only for bilateral breast implants.

Shortly thereafter, patient WC began her nutritional regimen. Initially, she suffered a several month period of migratory aches and pains, particularly severe in the right shoulder and hip, but these gradually resolved. She has now completed 18 months on her protocol, is in excellent health with no complaints. In fact, she has been feeling so well that after a prolonged period of disability, she has been able to resume work as a teacher.

Bone scans performed May 1, 1992—five months after patient WC began her treatment with me—and June 21, 1993 showed no evidence of metastatic disease. The earlier noted lesions had completely resolved.

Dr. Gonzalez presented these 25 cancer case studies to the NCI in 1993 and then updated the patient status information in 2001. Below are Dr. Gonzalez's personal notes with updated survival information:

Metastatic breast cancer. Alive and well. No sign of disease 9 years out. This patient's survival status was updated again in 2016. Please refer to page 257 for this additional information.

THOMAS JEFFERSON UNIVERSITY HOSPITA

CLINICAL LABORATORIES
DIRECTOR, REX B. CONN, M.D.

SURGICAL PATHOLOGY REPORT

Obtained on: 11/13/91
Accessioned: 11/13/91
Reported: 11/18/91
Physician: ANNE L ROSENBERG, MD
Service: SURGICAL
Location: JSC / NU : JSC

W   ,C
Med rec # :
Sex: F Age: 52
DOB: .   /39
Encounter# :
Surgical # : S91-

Source of Specimen:
    Part 1: BASE OF WOUND
    Part 2: LATERAL
    Part 3: SUPERIOR
    Part 4: MEDIAL
    Part 5: INFERIOR
    Part 6: RIGHT BREAST AT 6 O CLOCK

Clinical History and Diagnosis:
Right mass with calcification on mammography. 2nd cluster of
calcifications 1 cm away. Please R/O multicentric disease.

Frozen Section Diagnosis:
PART #1. A frozen section is received and read as "Infiltrating
ductal carcinoma", by Dr. Gibas

Gross Description:[G. Gibbons M.D./MMF]
PART #1. The specimen is labeled "Base of wound". It is
received fresh and consists of a single piece of fibrofatty tissue
measuring 0.5 cm in greatest dimension. The specimen is submitted in
its entirety into one cassette in a tissue bag.

Summary of sections:
1. undesignated, 1

PART #2. The specimen is labeled "Lateral". It is received fresh
and consists of fibrofatty tissue measuring 0.8 cm in greatest
dimension. The specimen is submitted in its entirety into one
cassette.

Summary of sections:
1. undesignated, 1

PART #3. The specimen is labeled "Superior". It is received fresh
and consists of a single piece of fibrofatty tissue measuring 1.0 x
0.9 x 0.6 cm. The specimen is submitted in its entirety into one
cassette.

Summary of sections:
1. undesignated, 1

1
--CONTINUED--

THOMAS JEFFERSON UNIVERSITY HOSPITA

CLINICAL LABORATORIES
DIRECTOR, REX B. CONN, M.D.

SURGICAL PATHOLOGY REPORT

W   .C   S91-

___

Gross Description (continued):

PART 4.   The specimen is labeled "Medial". It is received fresh and consists of a single piece of fibrofatty tissue measuring 0.8 x 0.7 x 0.6 cm. The specimen is submitted in its entirety into one cassette.

Summary of sections:
1. undesignated. 1

PART #5.   The specimen is labeled "Inferior". It is received fresh and consists of a single piece of fibrofatty tissue measuring 1.0 x 0.8 x 0.5 cm. The specimen is submitted in its entirety into one cassette.

Summary of sections:
1. undesignated. 1

PART #6.   The specimen is labeled "6 o'clock - right breast". It is received in fresh and measures 3.0 x 2.5 x 1.5 cm and also contains a needle and a single staple. A mammogram accompanies the specimen and shows a single discreet mass containing microcalcifications as well as multiple calcifications which are approximately 1 cm away from the above mentioned mass. The remainder of the specimen which has not been frozen is serially sectioned and submitted in its entirety into three cassettes. The remainder of the frozen sectioned was sent for ER/PR receptors. The specimen is inked.

Summary of sections:
3, undesignated, multiple

FINAL DIAGNOSIS: ***

1.   BREAST, BASE OF WOUND (BIOPSY):   NO TUMOR IDENTIFIED.

2.   BREAST, LATERAL (BIOPSY):   NO TUMOR IDENTIFIED.

3.   BREAST, SUPERIOR (BIOPSY):   NO TUMOR IDENTIFIED.

4.   BREAST, MEDIAL (BIOPSY):   NO TUMOR IDENTIFIED.

5.   BREAST, INFERIOR (BIOPSY):   NO TUMOR IDENTIFIED.

2
--CONTINUED--

THOMAS JEFFERSON UNIVERSITY HOSPITA
CLINICAL LABORATORIES
DIRECTOR, REX B. CONN, M.D.

SURGICAL PATHOLOGY REPORT

W   ,C   S91-

FINAL DIAGNOSIS (cont.):

6. BREAST, RIGHT, 6 O'CLOCK (BIOPSY): IN SITU AND INFILTRATING DUCT
CARCINOMA. SEE NOTE.

Note:
THE TUMOR MEASURES 2.1 CM. IN GREATEST DIAMETER. THE NUCLEAR GRADE
IS HIGH. THE HISTOLOGIC GRADE IS MODERATE. THE IN SITU COMPONENT IS
COMEDO TYPE. VASCULAR SPACE INVOLVEMENT IS IDENTIFIED. INVOLVED
DUCTS ARE SEEN AWAY FROM THE MAIN TUMOR MASS, WHICH MAY ACCOUNT
FOR THE APPEARANCE OF MULTICENTRICITY. HOWEVER, THE TUMORS APPEAR
TO BE OF ONE HISTOLOGIC TYPE.

Peter A. McCue, M.D./NGX

****

3

ANNE L ROSENBERG, MD
SUITE 602 M.O.B.
1100 WALNUT STREET

SURGICAL PATHOLOGY LABORATORY
Director:
Gerald C. Finkel M.D.

THOMAS JEFFERSON UNIVERSITY HOSPITAL **NUCLEAR MEDICINE DIVISION**	NAME W , C
	ROOM/WARD POP
	MED. RECORD NO.:
	SEX DR. A. ROSENBERG DR. A. DELCONTE
	AGE
	Doctor

SCAN REPORT: BONE SCAN: 12/2/91   SCAN NO.
               PROCEDURE CODE: 78306
               HISTORY: Breast Malignancy
               ICD CODE: 174.9

IMPRESSION:

Abnormal increased uptake in the right proximal femur. Radiological correlation is recommended to differentiate solitary metastases, vs benign trauma or fracture.

COMMENT:

Following the intravenous administration of 20 mCi of 99m Tc MDP, a whole body bone scan was performed. There is increased tracer uptake at the right proximal femur, which could represent benign trauma such as fracture or early solitary bone metastases. Therefore, further evaluation with x-ray tomography or MRI examination is recommended. If x-ray study is negative, early metastases should be considered.

In addition, there is a mild increased uptake at the proximal right tibial fibular junction which most likely represents degenerative changes. Otherwise, the remainder of the bone scan demonstrates mild degenerative changes involving both shoulder joints.

DATE: 12/3/91   S. _____
                                                          im

FORM 0346-01 (Rev. 9/86)

DOCTOR'S COPY

BINDING MARGIN – DO NOT WRITE OR PRINT IN THIS SPACE

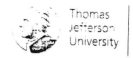

Thomas
Jefferson
University

| Jefferson Associates in Radiology | 111 South 11ᵀᴴ St |
| Consultation Report | Philadelphia, Pa. 19107 |

W.   . C   8915
OUTPATIENT   F52 (01/11/39)   MR

01/06/92 MRI EXTREMITIES/LOWER

ORDERED BY: Dr. Anne L Rosenberg

DIAGNOSIS:

Proximal right femoral lesion most likely representing a
metastatic focus although less likely representing an enchondroma.
Correlation with routine radiographs would be helpful.

COMMENT:

T1 & T2 axial, coronal and sagittal images of the right thigh were
performed with no previous studies available for comparison.

A solitary lesion is noted distal to the right greater trochanter
which is low on T1 and high on T2, most likely representing a
metastatic lesion although an enchondroma would be considered less
likely. There is minimal cortical involvement. The remaining
soft tissues and osseous structures appear unremarkable.

443.333

Dictated and signed: Mark Schweitzer, M.D./James T. Tsatalis, M.D.
Mailed: 01/06/92 2:11 pm

DR. NICHOLAS GONZALEZ   copies sent to:
737 PARK AVE   Dr. Anne L Rosenberg
NEW YORK,NY 10021   Dr. Anthony Delconte

Founded 1824

Jefferson Medical College · Thomas Jefferson University Hospital · College of Graduate Studies · College of Allied Health Sciences

64

NAME	W⋅⋅⋅⋅ ⋅ C⋅
ROOM/WARD	
MED. RECORD NO.:	POP
SEX	
AGE	DR. A. ROSENBERG
Doctor	

®

THOMAS JEFFERSON UNIVERSITY HOSPITAL
NUCLEAR MEDICINE DIVISION

SCAN REPORT: BONE SCAN: 5/1/92   SCAN NO.
PROCEDURE CODE:
HISTORY: Breast CA
ICD CODE: 174.9

IMPRESSION:

No definite evidence of metastatic disease.   No interval
change since 12/2/91.

COMMENT:

Following the intravenous administration of 20 mCi of 99m Tc
MDP, a whole body bone scan was performed.   Comparison is
made to a prior study of 12/2/91.   Again noted is mildly
increased uptake in the proximal right femur which remains
unchanged since the prior study.   Otherwise, there are no
areas of increased tracer uptake.   There is no definite
evidence of metastatic disease.

BINDING MARGIN – DO NOT WRITE OR PRINT IN THIS SPACE

DATE: ___4/30/91___   J. Greer/C. Intenzo,   M.D.

FORM 0346-01 (Rev. 9/86)   im

DOCTOR'S COPY

NAME	W C
ROOM/WARD	
MED. RECORD NO.:	POP
SEX	
AGE	
Doctor	DR. A. ROSENBERG DR. M. ARENA -1015 CHESNUT ST.

THOMAS JEFFERSON UNIVERSITY HOSPITAL
NUCLEAR MEDICINE DIVISION

Dr. Nicholas Gonzalez
737 Park Avenue
New York, N.Y. 10021

SCAN REPORT: SCAN NO.

BONE SCAN: 6/21/93
PROCEDURE CODE: 78306
HISTORY: BREAST CANCER
ICD CODE: 174.9

IMPRESSION:

No interval change and no evidence of metastatic disease.

COMMENT:

Following the intravenous administration of 25 mCi of 99m Tc MDP, a whole body bone scan was performed. Again there is no evidence of metastatic disease and there has been no interval change since the last examination dated 5/1/92.

BINDING MARGIN – DO NOT WRITE OR PRINT IN THIS SPACE

DATE: _____
4/22/93

_____ M.D.
C. Intenzo,

im

FORM 0346-01 (Rev. 9/86)

DOCTOR'S COPY

Uterine Cancer

8. Patient: LK
DOB: 8/11/44

Patient LK is a 48 year-old white female musician and horse trainer who felt well until the fall of 1990, when she required hospitalization for two episodes of deep venous thrombosis. She was placed on Coumadin, but shortly thereafter suffered an episode of severe endometrial hemorrhage. On December 24, 1990, because of bleeding, she underwent a D&C. Pathology studies documented endometrial carcinoma, and at St. Joseph's Hospital in Albuquerque she underwent a total abdominal hysterectomy with bilateral salpingo-oophorectomy.

Pathological examination showed endometrial adenocarcinoma with areas of squamous differentiation, high nuclear grade (FIGO grade III), involving the endometrium with 1/2 penetration of the myometrium and the superior portion of the endocervical canal, the left ovary, and obliterating the fimbriated end of the left Fallopian tube. Biopsies of the peritoneal cul de sac and the rectal serosa were positive for tumor implants. She was given a very poor prognosis.

Postoperatively, patient LK refused both chemotherapy and radiation, instead deciding to "take my chances." An abdominal MRI on March 3, 1991 showed periaortic adenopathy with persistent evidence of matted periaortic lymph nodes. Pelvic MRI on that date revealed diffuse pelvic adenopathy and evidence of pelvic mass lesion most notable in the left hemipelvis.

About that time, patient LK learned of my work and decided to pursue my therapy. She was first evaluated in my office on April 25, 1991. At that time, she reported feeling quite weak, with weight loss, malaise, night sweats and severe hot flashes. She was taking Sinequan QHS PRN and Darvocet PRN. Her examination and blood work were unremarkable.

Patient LK began her nutritional protocol in May 1991 and has been compliant since that time. Follow-up MRI done on December 31, 1991 showed no change in the periaortic lymphadenopathy as compared with the study of March 19, 1991, but near complete resolution of the pelvic adenopathy and no appreciable residual mass lesion in the left hemipelvis.

An MRI of the abdomen and pelvis done on January 5, 1993 indicated no significant intrapelvic pathology and no periaortic adenopathy. At that time, the lesions had virtually completely resolved. A single focal area of abnormal signal was noted in the lateral aspect of the liver, but this was also present on a previous scan and felt most compatible with benign hemangioma.

When last contacted on May 28, 1993, patient LK remained on her protocol and was in excellent health except for her menopausal symptoms. Patient LK clearly has done well on her program, with total regression of disease within a year.

Dr. Gonzalez presented these 25 cancer case studies to the NCI in 1993 and then updated the patient status information in 2001. Below are Dr. Gonzalez's personal notes with updated survival information:

Metastatic uterine cancer. Alive and well. No sign of disease 9 years out. This patient's survival status was updated again in 2016. Please refer to page 257 for this additional information.

ST. JOSEPH HOSPITAL
ALBUQUERQUE, NEW MEXICO

NAME: L. , K   PATH NO. S91-

AGE: 46Y   DATE: 02/0 /91
SEX: F   SURGEON: RITCHER
BIRTHDATE: /44   PATHOLOGIST: KEITH, T
MR#:   ID#:
ROOM: 3018-2   ROUTE/STOP: 3-25

CLINICAL DIAGNOSIS: ADENOCARCINOMA OF ENDOMETRIUM

TISSUE SUBMITTED: LEFT TUBE AND OVARY,RIGHT TUBE AND OVARY WITH
UTERUS,SMALL BOWEL SEROSA, LEFT PELVIC LYMPH NODE, RIGHT PELVIC LYMPH
NODE, PERITONEAL CUL DE SAC, RECTAL SEROSA, OMENTUM

GROSS DESCRIPTION: Specimen A is designated "left tube and ovary".
Received is a papillary tumor mass which lies adjacent to the
fimbriated end of the fallopian tube and adjacent to the ovary. The
entire mass measures 7x5.5x3 cm. The fallopian tube appears to end
abruptly in the mass. Sections from the tumor are submitted
designated T. Section of the tumor as the tube enters it is
designated TF. The tumor on frozen section shows adenocarcinoma,
probably endometrioid (TK). Frozen section control is submitted.
Sections from the fallopian tube are submitted designated F. Tumor
joins the surface of the ovary or appears to arise from the ovarian
stroma. Sections taken from the junction of the tumor and the ovary
are submitted designated TO.

Specimen B is designated "right tube and ovary and uterus". Received
is a uterus with adjacent fallopian tube and ovary. The right tube
and ovary are removed from the specimen and the uterus is weighed.
The uterus weighs 128 gm. The uterus measures 9x5x4 cm. The cervix
measures 2.5 cm. across with the cervical os of .3 cm. The uterus is
opened laterally revealing an endometrial cavity which is somewhat
enlarged and is lined by a nodular pink surface. On cross sectioning,
the surface is 6 to 8mm in depth. Grossly, the endometrium does not
appear to extend into the underlying myometrium. Sections of
endometrium are submitted designated E. Sections of the underlying
myometrium are submitted designated M. Two small rounded lesions are
present within the myometrium, both measuring 1 cm across. These
probably represent small leiomyomas. Bloody fluid is present within a
3mm. cystic space in the center of one of the leiomyomas. Sections of
cervix are submitted designated CA and CP corresponding to anterior
and posterior. Sections are also taken from the endocervical canal
extending up into the lower uterine segment. These sections are
designated ECA and ECP.

The right ovary measures 3x2x1.5 cm. The ovary is covered with reddish
pink membranous adhesions. On cross section, the ovary contains a 1
cm. cyst with a yellow inner lining. Sections of ovary are submitted
designated RO. The right fallopian tube measures 5 cm. in length and
1 cm. in greatest diameter. Sections from the fallopian tube are
submitted designated RF.

Specimen C is designated "small bowel serosa lesion for frozen
section". Received are four fragments of reddish gray tissue ranging
from 2 to 4mm in size. These fragments are submitted for frozen
section; frozen section shows granulation tissue (TK). Frozen section

PATHOLOGIST'S CONSULTATION REPORT

control is submitted.

Specimen D is designated "left pelvic lymph node". Received is a fragment of pinkish gray tan tissue measuring 1.5x1x.4 cm. The specimen is cross sectioned and is submitted in toto.

Specimen E is designated "right pelvic node". Received is a portion of tan tissue measuring 1x.5x.5 cm. Tissue fragment is cross sectione and is submitted in toto.

Specimen F is designated "peritoneal cul de sac biopsy". Received is a fragment of reddish gray tissue measuring 5x5x3mm. The specimen is cross sectioned and is submitted in toto.

Specimen G is designated "rectal serosa". Received is a fragment of reddish gray tissue measuring 15x2x2 mm. The fragment is submitted i toto.

Specimen H is designated "small bowel serosa". Received are small fragments of pinkish gray tissue which in aggregate measure 1x.5x.2 cm. These fragments are placed between sponges and are submitted in toto.

Specimen I is designated "omentum". Received is a portion of thin membranous omentum. The omentum measures 45x7x.5 cm. Mass lesions are not seen. Sections of omentum are submitted designated I.
TKmw

MICROSCOPIC DESCRIPTION: Numerous microscopic sections from the ovarian tumor show an adenocarcinoma with a mixed histologic pattern. In areas, the carcinoma forms back to back neoplastic glands lined by columnar cells with an endometrioid appearance. In other areas, these neoplastic cells form sheets and in focal areas show squamous - differentiation. The neoplastic cells are characterized by oval, hyperchromatic nuclei with dispersed nuclear chromatin and nucleoli and moderate to abundant amounts of eosinophilic cytoplasm. Mitoses are present and range from 0 to 3 mitoses per high power field. Other portions of the tumor have a papillary appearance with sheets of cells surrounding central fibrovascular core. The micropapillary projections from the papillary surfaces and the marked nuclear atypia is consistent with a papillary serous carcinoma. The carcinoma does not arise from fallopian tube epithelium. Tumor involves approximately one-half of the ovary.

Microscopic sections of cervix show normal appearing squamous epithelium and endocervical columnar epithelium. Areas of squamous metaplasia are noted. Sections from the endocervical canal show involvement of the upper portion of the endocervical canal by endometrial adenocarcinoma. In some sections, adenocarcinoma is present within the endocervical myometrium deep to surface endcervical glands. The carcinoma present within the upper portion of the endocervical canal and lower uterine segment is similar to that seen in the endometrium. In sections taken of the lower uterine segment, carcinoma extends into the myometrium to a distance of 1/2 myometrial wall thickness.

Numerous sections of endometrium show involvement by endometrial

PATHOLOGIST'S CONSULTATION REPORT

Proof of Concept

NAME: L. K.   PATH NO. S91-   Page

adenocarcinoma. The adenocarcinoma shows both a glandular and solid
growth pattern. Focal areas of squamous differentiation are also
identified. Nuclear atypia however is notable with the neoplastic
cells containing oval, hyperchromatic nuclei with dispersed chromatin
and prominent nucleoli. Sheets and columns of neoplastic cells exter
into the myometrium for a distance of 1/2 myometrial wall thickness.
In addition to carcinomatous involvement of myometrium, the myometriu
also demonstrates marked adenomyosis.

Sections from the right ovary show normal appearing ovarian stroma
containing multiple corpora albicantia. Tumor is not seen. Sections
from the right fallopian tube are also microscopically unremarkable.

Microscopic section from specimen C shows a portion of fibrovascular
tissue lined by mesothelium. Scattered acute and chronic inflammator
cells are noted. Tumor is not seen.

Microscopic section from specimen D shows a lymph node with
preservation of normal nodal architecture. Tumor is not identified.

Microscopic section from specimen E shows a lymph node which is
negative for tumor.

Microscopic section from specimen F shows a fragment of fibrovascular
tissue and granulation tissue with a mesothelial reaction. One small
clump of tumor consisting of a neoplastic gland is embedded within the
granulation tissue.

Microscopic section from specimen G shows a portion of granulation
tissue with a mesothelial proliferation and numerous scattered
polymorphonuclear leukocytes. Embedded within the granulation tissue
is a fragment of carcinoma. Several other scattered deposits of
single neoplastic cells and clusters of neoplastic cells are
identified within the granulation tissue.

Microscopic section from specimen H shows fragments of granulation
tissue with a mesothelial reaction and scattered acute inflammatory
cells. Definite carcinoma is not seen.

Microscopic section from specimen I show portions of adipose tissue.
The surface of the omentum shows a mesothelial reaction with scattered
acute and chronic inflammatory cells. Tumor is not seen.

DIAGNOSIS: A. Left tube and ovary: MIXED PAPILLARY SEROUS
                CARCINOMA AND ENDOMETRIOID CARCINOMA WITH
                AREAS OF SQUAMOUS DIFFERENTIATION. HIGH
                NUCLEAR GRADE (FIGO GRADE 3). TUMOR INVOLVES
                OVARY AND OBLITERATES FIMBRIATED END OF
                FALLOPIAN TUBE.

            B. Uterus, right tube and ovary:
                Cervix: MILD CHRONIC CERVICITIS.
                Endocervix: ENDOMETRIAL ADENOCARCINOMA
                    INVOLVES SUPERIOR PORTION OF ENDOCERVICAL
                    CANAL.

PATHOLOGIST'S CONSULTATION REPORT

72

NAME: L   K   PATH NO. S91-   Page 4

Endometrium: ENDOMETRIAL ADENOCARCINOMA WITH
    AREAS OF SQUAMOUS DIFFERENTIATION AND HIGH
    NUCLEAR GRADE (FIGO GRADE 3).
Myometrium: CARCINOMATOUS INVASION OF MYOMETRIUM
    TO 1/2 MYOMETRIAL WALL THICKNESS. ADENOMYOSIS
    (MARKED).
Right ovary and fallopian tube: NEGATIVE FOR
    TUMOR.

C. Small bowel serosal lesion: NEGATIVE FOR TUMOR.

D. Left pelvic lymph node: NEGATIVE FOR TUMOR.

E. Right pelvic lymph node: NEGATIVE FOR TUMOR.

F. Peritoneal cul-de sac, biopsy: SMALL TUMOR IMPLANTS
    WITH SURROUNDING GRANULATION TISSUE AND MESOTHELIAL
    REACTION.

G. Rectal serosa, biopsy: TUMOR IMPLANTS WITH
    SURROUNDING GRANULATION TISSUE AND MESOTHELIAL
    REACTION.

H. Small bowel serosa: GRANULATION TISSUE. NEGATIVE
    FOR TUMOR.

I. Omentum: MESOTHELIAL REACTION WITH ACUTE AND
    CHRONIC INFLAMMATION. NEGATIVE FOR TUMOR.

THOMAS KEITH, M.D.

QA: M
TK/RML:mw
02/09/91

SAN JUAN REGIONAL MEDICAL CENTER
FARMINGTON, NEW MEXICO
DEPARTMENT OF RADIOLOGY AND NUCLEAR MEDICINE
CONSULTATION REPORT

FAMILY NAME L.	K.	FIRST NAME	MIDDLE NAME		ROOM NO OP	1134-91
				SEX F	AGE YEARS 46	
REQUESTING PHYSICIAN DR. DUELGE				DATE OF STUDY 03-19-91		D

HISTORY

REPORT:

ABDOMINAL MR:

Images were obtained in multiple planes using various pulse sequences at SJR MR Center. Compared to the CT scan of 1/25/91, there has been decrease in degree of periaortic lymphadenopathy with persistent evidence of matted lymph nodes present most notable adjacent to the mid-pole of both kidneys. There is no evidence of abdominal ascites. The visualized liver appears enlarged, however, there is no definite evidence of metastatic disease. The spleen and both kidneys appear normal. There is no evidence of ascites. The visualized bony structures appear within normal limits.

CONCLUSION:

1. Interval improvement in degree of lymphadenopathy with persistent evidence of matted periaortic lymph nodes.
2. Findings of mild hepatomegaly.

MR OF PELVIS:

Images were obtained in multiple planes using various pulse sequences at SJR MR Center. Compared to the CT scan of 1/25/91, there is decrease in the degree of diffuse pelvic lymphadenopathy although there is persistent evidence of pelvic mass lesion most notable in the left hemipelvis. There is evidence of surgical defect presumably from previous hysterectomy. No definite free fluid is present within the pelvis, and all visualized bony structures are normal.

CONCLUSION:

Interval improvement in degree of diffuse adenopathy.

LANCE R. DELL, M.D.
03-26-91

rr
10:30 a.m.

FORM NO. _____ 8-87

SIGNATURE OF RADIOLOGIST

74

SAN JUAN REGIONAL MEDICAL CENTER
FARMINGTON, NEW MEXICO
DEPARTMENT OF RADIOLOGY AND NUCLEAR MEDICINE
CONSULTATION REPORT

..LY NAME	FIRST NAME	MIDDLE NAME		ROOM NO.	
...	K ...			OP	1134-91
			SEX	AGE - YEARS	
			F	47	

..UESTING PHYSICIAN	DATE OF STUDY	
DR. GONZALEZ	12-31-91	D

..ORY

..ORT

ABDOMINAL MR:

Images were obtained in multiple planes using various pulse sequences at San Juan Regional MR Center. Compared to the study of 3-19-91, degree of periaortic lymph adenopathy has not significantly changed. There definitely has been no significant increase in degree of adenopathy. There is no evidence of abdominal ascites. There has been slight interval decrease in overall size of the liver. The liver remains of homogenous, normal appearance. The visualized kidneys, pancreas and spleen also remain of homogenous, normal signal.

CONCLUSION:

No significant interval change in degree of periaortic lymph adenopathy.

MR PELVIS:

Images were obtained in multiple planes using various pulse sequences at San Juan Regional MR Center. Compared to the study of 3-19-91, there is continued improvement with near complete resolution of previously seen pelvic lymph adenopathy. Currently, there is no appreciable residual mass lesion present within the left hemipelvis and no free fluid within the pelvis. Previously described postoperative changes appear stable. Visualized bony structures show no significant abnormalities.

CONCLUSION:

Interval improvement in the appearance of the pelvis as above described.

LANCE A. DELL, M. D.
12-31-91

lft
7:30a.m.

FORM NO. E522032 (8/87)

SIGNATURE OF RADIOLOGIST ,

SAN JUAN REGIONAL MEDICAL CENTER
SAN JUAN REGIONAL MEDICAL CENTER RADIOLOGY & NUCLEAR MED
FARMINGTON, N.M.   Exam: 01/05/1993

NAME: ⬚ K   SEX: HOSP # . . .   PAT TYPE: OP

ORD DR: DR.   MISC. DOCTOR *Nickolas*   SS# 999-99-9999   DOB: . . . 1944
ATT DR: DR.   MISC. DOCTOR *Gonzales*
PATIENT ID: RM #   PROC: 72196   N MRPVS   PELVIS   AGE: 48

REASON:

MR OF THE PELVIS:

Images were obtained in multiple planes using various pulse
sequences at San Juan Regional MR Center. The current study is
compared to that of 12/31/91. There currently is no evidence of
significant pelvic mass. There is no identified pelvic
lymphadenopathy. No free fluid is present within the pelvis.
There is apparent surgical absence of the uterus. The visualized
bony structures are of homogeneous, normal signal.

CONCLUSION;

No significant intrapelvic pathology is demonstrated.

MR OF THE LIVER:

Images were obtained in multiple planes using various pulse
sequences at San Juan Regional MR Center. The current study is
compared to that of 12/31/91. There is evidence of a single focal
area of abnormal signal present in the lateral aspect of the right
lobe of the liver. Although this is not imaged in the study in
December of 1991, this is present in the study of 3/19/91. This
does present at a well circumscribed lesion with smooth peripheral
margins. There is decreased signal in T1 weighted imaging with
increased signal in T2 weighted imaging. The liver otherwise is of
homogeneous, normal signal. There is no evidence of significant
periaortic or periportal lymphadenopathy. There is no ascites.
The lung bases appear clear. The visualized bony structures are of
homogeneous, normal signal.

CONCLUSION:

The described finding in the right lobe of the liver is most
compatible with benign hemangioma. However, continued follow up
examinations are warranted.

Page 1

PRELIMINARY COPY

PHYSICIAN COPY 1

522032

ι .ι   ..   ٠...   ι_ฺ   .
                                                                                                        —

                         SAN JUAN REGIONAL MEDICAL CENTER
              SAN JUAN REGIONAL MEDICAL CENTER RADIOLOGY & NUCLEAR MED
                             FARMINGTON, N.M.   01/05/1993

NAME: L   K.   SEX: HOSP # ₂.₅₆(PAT TYPE: OP

DOCTOR: DR.   MISC. DOCTOR   SS#   DOB: '1944

PATIENT ID: ₁₃₃₄₃₁   RM #   PROC: 72196   N MRPVS   PELVIS   AGE: 48

REASON:

                              (Page 2)

                                        LANCE A. DELL, M.D.
                                        01-14-93
      jlw

01/14/1993 17:49:09

                              PRELIMINARY COPY

                         PHYSICIAN COPY 1   522032 (7/92)
                                                                     _____

Head and Neck Cancer

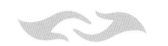

9. Patient: GB
DOB: 6-10-48

Patient GB is a 45 year-old white woman who had been in excellent health when in the spring of 1989, she developed an enlarged cervical node. She was otherwise asymptomatic. A needle biopsy in July 1989 was negative. However, the node continued to enlarge and on May 23, 1990, patient GB underwent an excisional biopsy that revealed metastatic poorly differentiated squamous cell carcinoma with minute foci of keratinization replacing lymph node. CT scan of head and neck on June 1, 1990 showed a small nodule projecting from the base of the tongue on the right side, but no definite adenopathy. A subsequent biopsy of the tongue lesion on June 5, 1990 documented a small area of superficially invasive squamous cell carcinoma in a background of severe squamous dysplasia. Radiation and surgery were recommended, but adamantly refused by patient GB.

Patient GB instead decided to pursue my therapy, and was first seen in my office on July 12, 1990. At that time, she had no complaints, was on no medications, and had an unremarkable physical examination except for a right tongue lesion.

Patient GB has been a very compliant patient, except for a period of hospitalization after an automobile accident in July 1990. She has completed three years on her protocol, currently lives in Colorado, appears to be completely disease free and is in excellent health. She would seem to be a very unusual patient who has survived with a metastatic head and neck malignancy.

Dr. Gonzalez presented these 25 cancer case studies to the NCI in 1993 and then updated the patient status information in 2001. Below are Dr. Gonzalez's personal notes with updated survival information:

Metastatic head and neck cancer. Alive and well 10 years out.

Diagnostic Radiology Associates

FACULTY PRACTICE

| Diagnostic Radiology & Nuclear Medicine
Suite 522
(212) 242-7307 - (212) 242-7308 | 36 Seventh Avenue
NEW YORK, N.Y. 10011 | Ultrasound & Computerized Tomography
Suite 408
(212) 242-7362 - (212) 242-7851 |

June 1, 1990

Robert C. Eberle, M.D.
130 West 12th Street
New York, N.Y.   10011

RE: G   , B

Dear Dr. Eberle:

CT SCAN OF HEAD & NECK   6/1/90

Scans were obtained from the base of the skull through the clavicles. There is a small polypoid excrescence projecting into the left antrum from the medial wall.

There is a small nodule projecting from the base of the tongue on the right, into the vallecular area. This is seen on image 21 of the upper series. No definite adenopathy is noted in the upper neck, either on the right side or on the left side.

Scans of the lower neck through the level of the clavicular heads, show no abnormalities.

Thank you for referring this patient.

Sincerely yours,

Lawrence Zingesser, M.D.

LZ/ajd

ST. VINCENT'S HOSPITAL
AND MEDICAL CENTER OF NEW YORK
DEPARTMENT OF PATHOLOGY

PATHOLOGY NO.   90 4467

DATE   5/23/90   3:18 pm

CHART NO.

NAME   G , B   HALL   PA   AGE   41

DIVISION   Surgery   SURGEON   Dr. Eberle

TISSUE   Lymph node neck

FROZEN SECTION DIAGNOSIS: Metastatic, poorly differentiated, squamous cell
carcinoma with microscopic foci of keratinization.

I. TOTH, M.D., PATHOLOGIST

HISTORY

Susp. on Cytology for lymphoma several mos. ago.

CLINICAL DIAGNOSIS   Lymphoma

PATHOLOGICAL REPORT

The specimen is labeled lymph node neck and is received fresh for
Frozen Section. See Above. The specimen consists of a single, irregular, soft
tissue fragment, measuring 3.5 x 2 x 1 cm in greatest dimensions. The outer
surface is dark-red and hemorrhagic appearing. The cut surface displays a
white-tan, as well as a pink-red aspect. The former also displays areas which
are white-tan and chaulky appearing. The specimen is entirely submitted in
five (5) cassettes labeled FSA, A1, A2, A3 and A4.   MK/mf

MICROSCOPIC DIAGNOSIS: 8143⁴

FSA, A1 - A3:   Lymph node biopsy of neck for frozen section:

Metastatic poorly differentiated squamous cell carcinoma with minute foci
of keratinization replacing lymph node.
There is no evidence of malignant lymphoma.

NOTE: The site of origin cannot be determined in histological grounds.
Clinical studies are helpful.

PATHOLOGIST

I. TOTH, M.D.   5/25/90   mf

ST. VINCENT'S HOSPITAL
AND MEDICAL CENTER OF NEW YORK
DEPARTMENT OF PATHOLOGY

PATHOLOGY NO.

DATE 6/ 1   10:27

CHART NO.

NAME G.... X.....   LOC.   AGE 41/F

DEPARTMENT Surgery   M.D. Eberle
                             CC:

TISSUE Base tongue, right side

HISTORY   ...see card

CLINICAL DIAGNOSIS

Carcinoma

PATHOLOGICAL REPORT

Specimen labeled "base tongue, right side" is received in formalin. Specimen consists of multiple fragments of tan-brown, focally hemorrhagic tissue admixed with soft yellow lobulated tissue measuring .3x.4x.1cm. in aggregate. Specimen entirely submitted in lens paper in one cassette.

XL/wc

MICROSCOPIC DIAGNOSIS: 1073

Multiple fragments of squamous mucosa with adjacent lymphoid tissue showing focal small area of superficially invasive squamous cell carcinoma in a background of severe squamous dysplasia.

NOON NY LEE, M.D.   PATHOLOGIST
                           6/2/90 wc

84-225S-REV. 5/89 P-5/89

Lung Cancer

10. Patient: DD
DOB: 3/4/29

Patient DD is a 64 year-old white male with a history of adenoid cystic carcinoma of the trachea with metastases to the lung. Patient DD has a history of cigar smoking, but had been in good health when he developed the sensation of a nodule on the left side of his throat in 1977. His physician thought the symptoms were insignificant, and no diagnostic tests were pursued. Over the following three years, the nodule gradually increased in size. When patient DD developed wheezing and dyspnea on exertion, he returned to his physician who told him he had emphysema and arthritis of the neck. When the symptoms worsened he was referred to a pulmonologist who suspected a chronic infection and prescribed various antibiotics and other medications for a period of a year, with no effect. Finally, patient DD was referred for a CT of the trachea on June 12, 1981, which revealed a large tumor of the tracheal wall at the level of the thoracic inlet. Patient DD was referred in turn to a surgeon and on June 17, 1981 at New York University he underwent transcervical and transthoracic resection of the trachea with primary anastomosis and suprahyoid laryngeal release. Pathological examination showed adenoid cystic carcinoma. He subsequently received 6000 rads to the tumor bed.

Patient DD did well until November 1987, when a routine chest X-ray demonstrated multiple pulmonary nodules. A needle biopsy of a lesion on December 29, 1987 revealed metastatic adenoid cystic carcinoma. At that time, his doctors said he might live another six months to a year.

Patient DD learned of my work, and was first seen in my office on May 3, 1988. At that time, he had no complaints and was on no medications. His examination was notable only for psoriasis.

He began his nutritional protocol soon after seeing me and has continued on it to this time. In general, he has been a determined and compliant patient except for dietary lapses. When last seen in late 1992, he was in excellent health, enjoying his retirement, fully active and denying any respiratory or systemic symptoms.

About every 12 months, patient DD has a chest X-ray: the studies show, according to the formal reports, gradual "progression of disease," but I suspect the films reveal not worsening cancer, but fibrotic change around the tumors. This is not an uncommon finding in my patients. Furthermore, since the median survival for metastatic adenoid cystic carcinoma is nine months, patient DD, whatever the X-rays show, is certainly an unusual patient.

Dr. Gonzalez presented these 25 cancer case studies to the NCI in 1993 and then updated the patient status information in 2001. Below are Dr. Gonzalez's personal notes with updated survival information:

Recurrent lung cancer. Alive and well 12 years out. This patient's survival status was updated again in 2016. Please refer to page 257 for this additional information.

University Radiology Associates, P.C.

New York Medical College
Valhalla, New York 10595

DIAGNOSTIC RADIOLOGY
MICHAEL S. TENNER, M.D., F.A.C.R.   SUSAN FREEMAN, M.D.   DENISE LESLIE, M.D.
RITA F. GIROLAMO, M.D., F.A.C.R.   GRACE GEORGE, M.D.   ALEX NORMAN, M.D., F.A.C.R.
ROBERT M. KLEIN, M.D., F.A.C.R.   LOUISE GODINE, M.D.   PAUL SANE, M.D.
HOWARD BERMAN, M.D.   STUART KATZ, M.D.   ANDREW SCHECHTER, M.D.
JOSEPH R. FAKHRY, M.D.   SUSAN KLEIN, M.D.   MICHAEL SWIRSKY, M.D.

RADIATION MEDICINE
BASIL S. HILARIS, M.D., F.A.C.R.
CHITTI R. MOORTHY, M.D.
MICHAEL S. PORRAZZO, M.D.
ANCA E. TCHELEBI, M.D.

TELEPHONES
BUSINESS OFFICE   914-347-3589
OP REGISTRATION   914-285-1452
MACY X-RAY   914-285-7341
MUNGER X-RAY   914-993-4377

May 10, 1990

Dr. N. Gonzalez
737 Park Avenue
New York, New York 100211 Center

RE: D   , C . .

Dear Dr. Gonzalez:

Thank you for referring the above patient for examination performed on 5/9/90.

CHEST: Two projections: No clinical history is indicated on the requisition form. There is evidence of metastatic diseae which appears to have increased both in number and size. This is in comparison to earlier study of 4/21/89.

Sincerely,

M. H. Swirsky, M.D.

mhs;ac
DD: 5/9/90
DT: 5/9/90

MEDICAL CENTER.   REPORT OF EXAMINATION   LAB NO.   0419-01
UNIVERSITY HOSPITAL   OF TISSUE

NAME OF PATIENT				UNIT NO.	ROOM
D. D.					1204

SEX	AGE	DATE SPECIMEN		DATE OF REPORT	COPIES	
		TAKEN	RECEIVED			
M	52	June 17, 1981	June 19, 1981	June 25, 1981		

DOCTOR	NATURE OF SPECIMEN TAKEN
N. Cohen, M.D. ✓ A. Boyd, M.D.	1. Trachea. 2. Inferior margin of trachea. 3. Trachea. 4. Trachea cartilage. 5. Trachea tumor.

FINAL DIAGNOSIS

1. Trachea: Fragment of respiratory mucosa with chronic inflammation, No tumor seen.
2. Inferior margin of trachea: Adenoid cystic carcinoma in smooth muscle and accessory mucus glands.
3. Trachea: Segment of trachea infiltrated by adenoid cystic carcinoma.
4. Trachea cartilage: Segment of trachea infiltrated by adenoid cystic carcinoma.
5. Trachea tumor: Large segment of trachea including tracheostomy site infiltrated by adenoid cystic carcinoma. Tracheostomy site free of tumor.   (M)

                                    E. Fenchel, M.D. / G. Valensi, M.D.

FROZEN SECTION DIAGNOSES: 1- Respiratory mucosa, no tumor seen. (E. Fazzini, M.D.)
                            2- Adenoid cystic carcinoma in respiratory mucosa.
                               (E. Fazzini, M.D.)
                            3- Adenoid cystic carcinoma in respiratory mucosa.
                               (E. Fazzini, M.D.)

MACROSCOPIC EXAMINATION:

The specimen is received in five parts.

Part 1 is labelled "trachea." Part 2 is labelled "trachea." Part 3 is labelled "inferior margin of trachea." Part 4 is labelled "tracheal cartilage." Part 5 is labelled "tracheal tumor." Specimens 1 through 4 are received in the fresh state.

Specimen #1 consists of a fragment of cartilage and soft tissue measuring 4 mm. in diameter. The entire specimen is submitted for frozen section diagnosis and labelled "A."

Specimen #2 consists of an irregular fragment of soft tissue and cartilage measuring 6 mm. in diameter. The entire specimen is submitted for frozen section study and labelled "B."

Specimen #3 consists of a segment of cartilage which is linear and measures 1 cm. in length. One-half of the specimen is submitted for frozen section study and labelled "C." The remainder is submitted labelled "D."

CONTINUED ON PAGE TWO .

```
11/21/87 09:41 PM              PAGE 004
```

```
| | | | | | | | | | | | | | | | | | | |
    D.  D              DSCH
   0616514  91529  03/04/29  58   M
   JACOBS JOSEPH MD
| | | | | | | | | | | | | | | | | | | | | | | | | | | | | | | |
```

ANCILLARY RESULTS:
= = = = = = = = =

I-314-248 04:31 AM 11/12/87   INTERPRETER: STAIGER, MELINDA
   9.01 EXAMINATION PERFORMED:11/10/87

        RESULTS FOR: PST CHEST PA/LT LATERAL

        MIDLINE STERNAL SUTURE IS NOTED ANTERIORLY. THERE IS APPARENT
        WIDENING OF THE SUPERIOR MEDIASTINUM, POSSIBLY SECONDARY TO
        ADENOPATHY AND CORRELATION WITH CHEST C.T. IS RECOMMENDED.
        BILATERAL VERY ROUND PULMONARY NODULES ARE NOTED, THE LARGEST
        BEING IN THE LUL. THESE ARE SUSPICIOUS METASTATIC NODULES AND
        CLINICAL CORRELATION IS RECOMMENDED. NO FOCAL INFILTRATE OR
        EFFUSION IS IDENTIFIED.

        DD 11/11/87
        11/11/87 LS

I-320-202 11:43 AM 11/18/87   INTERPRETER: STAIGER, MELINDA
  26.01 EXAMINATION PERFORMED:11/17/87 RESULTS FOR: C.T. CHEST

        MULTIPLE SEQUENTIAL AXIAL CUTS WERE OBTAINED FROM THE THORACIC
        INLET THROUGH THE HEMIDIAPHRAGMS AT 10 MM. INTERVALS WITHOUT
        INTRAVENOUS CONTRAST ADMINISTRATION.

        NO SIGNIFICANT AXILLARY OR MEDIASTINAL ADENOPATHY IS
        APPRECIATED. THERE IS FULLNESS OF BOTH HILAR REGIONS, HOWEVER,
        CONSISTENT WITH BILATERAL HILAR ADENOPATHY. IN ADDITION,
        BILATERAL PULMONARY NODULES, THE LARGEST OF WHICH MEASURES
        APPROXIMATELY 1 TO 1.5 CMS. IN DIAMETER AND IS SEEN IN THE
        LEFT UPPER LOBE ARE NOTED. THERE IS NO EVIDENCE OF FOCAL
        INFITLRATE OR EFFUSION. NO ENDOBRONCHIAL PATHOLOGY IS
        IDENTIFIED.

        IMPRESSION: BILATERAL HILAR ADENOPATHY IN ASSOCIATION WITH
        MULTIPLE PULMONARY NODULES BILATERALLY. THESE FINDINGS ARE
        SUSPICIOUS FOR EITHER INFECTIOUS OR NEOPLASTIC DISEASE AND
        CLINICAL CORRELATION IS RECOMMENDED. INCIDENTALLY NOTED IS
        EVIDENCE OF A SINGLE MIDLINE STERNAL SUTURE.

        IMPRESSION: BILATERAL HILAR ADENOPATHY ASSOCIATED WITH
        BILATERAL PULMONARY NODULES.

        DD/DT 11/18/87 PMG.

ALL CURRENT TEST AND DISCHARGE ORDERS

                                        CONTINUED
|||||||||||||||||||||||||||||||||||||||||||||||||||||||||||||||||||||||||||||||||||||
DEAN DONALD   TEST RESULTS SUMMARY
```
```

NEW YORK UNIVERSITY
MEDICAL CENTER
(212) 340-6455

CYTOPATHOLOGY

Physician Performing Procedure: Schlessberg
Telephone No.: 5439
Date Requested: 12/29/87

Return Report to Dr.: Boyd   Location: _   Tel.: 7287

294677 BNY 138SCC   61-65-14
BOYD ARTHUR MD
JACOBS JOSEPH MD
0616516 U3/04/29 M 58
12/28/87

IF OUT PATIENT NEED ADDRESS FOR BILLING

Date of Birth: Medicare No.:

GYN
SOURCE C V E
☐ ☐ ☐
☐ Other
Specify ___
No. of Slides ___

BRUSH
☐ Bronchial   ☐ Colonic
☐ Esophageal   ☐ Oral
☐ Gastric   Other
☐ Urinary Tract ☐ ___

NEEDLE ASPIRATIONS
☐ Breast ☐ Lymph ☐ Retroperitoneum
☐ Bone   Node   ☐ Pancreas
☐ CNS   ☐ Salivary ☐ Prostate
☑ Lung   Gland Other
☐ Liver ☐ Thyroid ☐ ___

FLUIDS
☐ Bronchial Wash   ☐ Ascitic   ☐ Voided Urine ☐ Esophageal Wash ☐ CSF   ☐ Pleural
☐ Bronchial Lavage ☐ Peritoneal Wash ☐ Cath. Urine ☐ Sputum ☐ LP   ☐ Breast
   ☐ Pericardial ☐ Bladder Wash ☐ Gastric Wash ☐ SHUNT Other
   ☐ Cysto Urine ☐ Nipple

CONSULT ☐   Log Number and Accession Date
From: NL-7465
   12-29-87 3:45 in
   out 3:00PM 12/30
Spec:
No. Slides: No. Slides 1 PAP, 2HE + CB

Clinical History and Source of Specimen:

Hx Ca Trachea 1981
Now - many nodules in lungs
R/O Mets

SEX ☐ M ☐ F   AGE   RACE   PREVIOUS CYTOLOGY ☐ No ☐ Yes   INPATIENT ☐   OUTPATIENT ☐

HISTORY
RADIATION	CHEMOTHERAPY	RECENT INSTRUMENTATION CYSTOSCOPY OR ENDOSCOPY:	RECENT SURGERY:	INFECTION BIOHAZARD RISK FACTOR	None	AIDS	IVDA	Hepatitis	TB	Other
☐ Yes ☐ No When:	☐ Yes ☐ No Specify:		When: Describe:							

ADDITIONAL GYN HISTORY
DATE OF SMEAR: LMP: PREVIOUS CYTOLOGY ☐ Yes ☑ No   IF YES, WHEN? CYTOLOGY RESULTS: IF BIOPSY, RESULTS:

PREGNANT	ABNORMAL BLEEDING	OB HISTORY G__ P__ Ab__	CONTRACEPTION ☐ IUD ☐ Pills ☐ Other	LEUCORRHEA	HORMONAL THERAPY
☐ Yes ☐ No	☐ Yes ☐ No			☐ Yes ☐ No	☐ Yes ☐ No
COLPOSCOPY ☐ Yes ☐ No	CRYOSURGERY ☐ Yes ☐ No	CAUTERY ☐ Yes ☐ No	RADIATION ☐ Yes ☐ No When?	CHEMOTHERAPY ☐ Yes ☐ No Specify:	HYSTERECTOMY ☐ Yes ☐ No OTHER SURGERY?

DO NOT WRITE BELOW THIS LINE.   FOR LABORATORY USE ONLY

CYTOLOGY REPORT — GYN ONLY
☐ Negative   ☐ Endometrial Cells Present   ☐ Repeat   ☐ Scanty Material
☐ Inflammation   ☐ Trichomonas   ☐ Inadequate for Diagnosis   ☐ Squamous Metaplasia
☐ Inflammatory Squamous Atypia ☐ Candida   ☐ Menstrual Smear Pattern ☐ Atrophic Smear Pattern
☐ Inflammatory Endocervical Atypia ☐ No Endocervical Component ☐ Blood Present   ☐ Radiation Effect

DESCRIPTION AND FINAL DIAGNOSIS:

Aspirate from lung:
Smears and cell block:
Positive for malignant cells.
Cellular specimen consisting of single atypical
cells and sheets of cells forming a cribriform
pattern. An acellular amorphous material fills the
cribriform spaces.
Diagnosis: Metastatic adenoid cystic carcinoma.

CYTOTECHNOLOGIST	DATE OF REPORT	PATHOLOGIST	SNOMED CODE(S)	TR CODE
12/31/87	12/31/87	Kathryn Hinnant M.D. 1-4-88		

Form No. Rev. 1/86

11. Patient: SA
DOB: 1/23/36

Patient SA was a 54 year-old white male with a history of metastatic adenocarcinoma of the lung who was lost to follow up in the fall of 1989 after enjoying significant improvement in his illness.

Patient SA had a long history of cigarette use. In early 1987, he first developed chest pain and cough, and went to his local physician for evaluation. After an X-ray revealed a right lung mass, on March 16, 1987, patient SA underwent bronchoscopy with biopsy which showed adenocarcinoma of the lung. Although surgery was immediately suggested, patient SA refused all treatment. However, when his symptoms worsened, he agreed to surgery and at Norwalk Hospital in July, 1987 he underwent a right pneumonectomy followed by a course of radiation (4500 rads) to the chest.

Patient SA subsequently did well until Sept 1988, when he developed headaches and pressure behind the right eye. After a CT scan of the head indicated lesions in the right frontal and right temporal lobe consistent with metastatic disease, patient SA completed a course of 3000 rads radiation therapy to the head, which he completed on November 9, 1988. Patient SA refused a course of suggested chemotherapy.

A CT scan of the abdomen at that time demonstrated evidence of left adrenal mass 4.4 cm. by 2.5 cm. felt consistent with metastatic disease. A bone scan showed positive areas, and a CT scan of the head from December 5, 1988—a month after patient SA completed radiation to the head—indicated progression of his brain disease despite treatment:

"Multiple, bilateral intracerebral ring-enhancing lesions, consistent with metastases. In addition there appears to be an early left cerebellar hemisphere lesion. Many of these were noted on 10/18/88. However, several new small areas of abnormality are identified on the present exam, not previously seen. This could either be due to progression of the metastatic disease versus improved visualization…"

Patient SA first presented to me on December 6, 1988. At that time, he reported fatigue and a recurrence of his headaches: he was on Decadron, Dilantin and Zantac. His examination was notable only for absent breath sounds consistent with his history.

Patient SA began his nutritional program in late December 1988, and noted an immediate improvement in his symptoms. Then on January 18, 1989, after patient SA had completed a month on his protocol, a CT scan showed definite improvement in his brain lesions:

"When compared to the last previous exam of 12/5/88, there has been diminution both in size and number of the visualized intracranial lesions. No new areas of abnormality are seen."

According to his oncologist's notes, a bone scan in March 1989 showed clearing of the previous lesions, and an abdominal CT scan revealed "No change in size of adrenal mass on CT."

At that time, patient SA was symptom-free and back to work full-time as draftsman. Unfortunately, he felt so well he became careless with his supplements and diet, and by April was by his own admission less than 50% compliant with his protocol. Not surprisingly, his neurological symptoms returned and a CT scan done May 1 1989 revealed somewhat worsening disease:

"Increased intracranial edema and size of previously reported intracranial metastases when compared to 3/7/89…"

After a stern lecture from me, patient SA became more compliant; his symptoms rapidly improved and a CT scan from July 2, 1989 demonstrated reduction in all this brain tumors:

"The three metastatic lesions on the 5/1/89 CT have decreased in size. No new metastatic lesions are seen…"

Unfortunately, with return of good health, patient SA again became careless with his protocol. I last saw him September 28, 1989: at that time, after several weeks of non-compliance, his neurological symptoms had returned. Thereafter, he was lost to follow-up. Unfortunately, he had no family that I knew of, and I have been unable to obtain the actual scans although I have all the written reports.

Patient SA represents an unfortunate, though interesting case because inadvertently he became his own control. While following his nutritional program completely, his brain lesions rapidly regressed: when off his protocol, the tumors quickly grew.

Dr. Gonzalez presented these 25 cancer case studies to the NCI in 1993 and then updated the patient status information in 2001. Below are Dr. Gonzalez's personal notes with updated survival information:

Metastatic lung cancer to brain and abdomen. Quit the program after enjoying significant regression, then lost to follow-up.

Aisle 3-Bay 2-846

Proof of Concept - 25 Best Cancer Case
Sku: 4JSHAO002JHM

Good

All pages and cover are intact - The book may have some
cosmetic wear (i.e. creased spine/cover, scratches,
curled corners, folded pages, minor sunburn) - The book
has very few or no highlight/notes/underlined pages -
Safe and Secure Mailer - No Hassle Return - Used books
may not include supplementary material.

Ship To

Mike Hamel
12192 SE 21st Avenue
Starke, FL 32091

Order Details

Order ID	661639586
Order Date	12/23/2022 8:01:35 PM
Shipping Service	Standard
Buyers Name	Mike Hamel

Rock Safe LLC strives to have each and
every customer 100% satisfied with
their purchase. If for any reason you
are not 100% satisfied please email us
at bookz1012@gmail.com with your
concerns.

If we need to make something right,
we will, Guaranteed!

Aisle 3 - Bay 2-846

Proof of Concept - 25 Best Cancer Case
Sku: 4JSHAO002JHM

Good

All pages and cover are intact - The book may have some cosmetic wear (i.e. creased spine, cover scratches, curled corners, folded pages, minor sunburn) - The book has very few or no highlight notes/underlined pages - Safe and Secure Mailer - No Hassle Return - Used books may not include supplementary material.

Ship To

Mike Hamel
12192 SE 21st Avenue
Starke, FL, 32091

Order Details

Order ID	66169686
Order Date	12/29/2022 8:01:25 PM
Shipping Service	Standard
Buyers Name	Mike Hamel

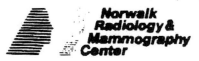

Norwalk Radiology & Mammography Center

148 East Avenue, Norwalk, CT 06851
(203) 838-4886

THOMAS W. VRIS, M.D.
ONE MOTT AVENUE
NORWALK, CT. 06851

DEAR DR. VRIS:

In reference to your recent referral of:

S. A.

10/19/88 15:00   CT HEAD W O. W CONTRAST OT SEC

Examination: CT of the Sinuses

CT of the sinuses shows the sinuses to be clear. The facial bones are intact.

Contrast enhanced CT of the head was then performed. Head CT shows in the right temporal region that there is a focus of ill defined contrast enhancement measuring approximately one to one and a half cm. in diameter which is surrounded by a significant amount of white matter edema.

A several mm. focus of contrast enhancement is seen in the right frontal lobe with surrounding white matter edema as well.

In the left occipital region there is an approximately 2 cm. in diameter ring enhancing lesion with surrounding edema.

IMPRESSION:

CT of the head shows evidence of brain metastases (right temporal, right frontal, and left occipital) with surrounding edema. There is no shift of midline structures or evidence of metastatic involvement of the facial bones or sinuses.

Thank you for referring Mr. A.   to our office

CHRIS MCGARY, M.D.

xCR: PAB/I

James S. Bauman, M.D. William T. Cronin, M.D. Alan H. Levine, M.D. Richard J. Lisi, M.D. Avelino N. Maitem, M.D.
Chris McGary, M.D. Pradip Pathare, M.D. Alan H. Richman, M.D. Tina S. Richman, M.D. Edward B. Strauss, M.D.

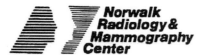

Norwalk Radiology & Mammography Center

148 East Avenue, Norwalk, CT 06851
(203) 838-4886

KESAVAN NAIR, M.D.   12/05/88
40 CROSS STREET
NORWALK, CT.   06851

DEAR DR. NAIR:

In reference to your recent referral of:

S. A   #4506

12/05/88 10:00   CT HEAD WITH CONTRAST

Examination: CT Scan Head

5 mm sections were obtained through the entire cranium, following
the administration of a double-dose of intravenous contrast. The
study was compared to 10/19/88.

Again noted are multiple, ring-enhancing intracranial lesions,
consistent with metastases. These are located bilaterally in the
right middle cranial fossa, left occipital region, (periatrial),
right temporal lobe, right frontal region, right parietal lobe
and the left paracentral partial-occipital region. In addition,
there appears to be a small ring-enhancing lesion in the left
cerebellar hemisphere. Many of these lesions were previously
noted, but several new lesions are identified on this exam that
were not seen on the previous exam. This could be due to either
progression of the disease versus improved visualization, due to
the double-dose of intravenous contrast. There is still evidence
of edema, most notably in the right temporal lobe and the left
parietal lobe.

IMPRESSION:

Multiple, bilateral intracerebral ring-enhancing lesions,
consistent with metastases. In addition, there appears to be an
early left cerebellar hemisphere lesion. Many of these were
noted on 10/18/88. However, several new, small areas of
abnormality are identified on the present exam, not previously
seen. This could either be due to progression of the metastatic
disease versus improved visualization, due to the use of a
double-dose of intravenous contrast.

Thank you for referring Mr. A   to our office

                                    JAMES BAUMAN, M.D.

COPY TO DR. PATHARE AND DR. GREENWALD

James S. Bauman, M.D. William T. Cronin, M.D. Alan H. Levine, M.D. Richard J. Lisi, M.D. Avelino N. Maitem, M.D.
Chris McGary, M.D. Pradip Pathare, M.D. Alan H. Richman, M.D. Tina S. Richman, M.D. Edward B. Strauss, M.D.

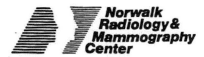

Norwalk Radiology & Mammography Center

148 East Avenue, Norwalk, CT 06851
(203) 838-4886

KESAVAN NAIR, M.D.   12/05/88
40 CROSS STREET
NORWALK, CT.   06851

DEAR DR. NAIR:

In reference to your recent referral of:

S. A

12/05/88 09:00   CT ABDOMEN WITH CONTRAST

Examination: CT Scan Abdomen

Contiguous sections were obtained through the abdomen following the administration of both intravenous and p.o. contrast. The study was compared to the most recent exam of 10/31/88.

Again noted is a right pleural effusion. The liver, spleen, pancreas, biliary system and kidneys are normal. There is no evidence of adenopathy or ascites. The right adrenal gland is normal.

Again noted is a left adrenal mass. This measures 4.4 cm x 2.5 cm. This is approximately equivalent to what it measured on 10/31/88.

IMPRESSION:

1. No significant interval change in the appearance of the left adrenal mass, measuring 4.4 cm x 2.5 cm. No new areas of abdominal pathology are identified.

2. Right pleural effusion.

Thank you for referring Mr. A   to our office

JAMES BAUMAN, M.D.

COPY TO DR. PATHARE AND DR. GREENWALD

XCR: ODE/I

James S. Bauman, M.D. William T. Cronin, M.D. Alan H. Levine, M.D. Richard J. Lisi, M.D. Avelino N. Maitem, M.D.
Chris McGary, M.D. Pradip Pathare, M.D. Alan H. Richman, M.D. Tina S. Richman, M.D. Edward B. Strauss, M.D.

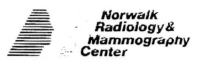

Norwalk Radiology & Mammography Center

148 East Avenue, Norwalk, CT 06851
(203) 838-4886

KESAVAN NAIR, M.D.   01/18/89
40 CROSS STREET
NORWALK, CT., '06851

DEAR DR. NAIR:

In reference to your recent referral of:

S. A.

01/18/89 09:00   CT HEAD WITH CONTRAST

Examination: CT Scan Head With Contrast

5 mm and 10 mm sections were obtained following the infusion of contrast and compared to the last previous exam of 12/5/88.

Still identified, but appearing improved, is the presence of intracerebral lesions involving the right frontal region, left occipital region and anterior right temporal region. These lesions were previously noted on the last previous exam and appeared larger and there was more evidence of vasogenic edema. There is still some evidence of low-density in the right temporal region and left occipital region, but this does appear improved from the last previous exam. Previously, several small, scattered ring-enhancing nodules were seen in both cerebral hemispheres. Many of these are not identified on the present exam. No new areas of abnormality are seen. There is no evidence of herniation or midline shift. No extra-axial fluid collections are seen.

IMPRESSION:

When compared to the last previous exam of 12/5/88, there has been diminution both in size and number of the visualized intracranial lesions. No new areas of abnormality are seen.

Thank you for referring Mr. A   to our office

JAMES BAUMAN, M.D.

XCR: ODE/I

James S. Bauman, M.D. William T. Cronin, M.D. Alan H Levine, M.D. Richard J. Lisi, M.D. Avelino N. Maitem, M.D.
Chris McGuire, M.D. Prudic Pathare, M.D. Alan H Richman, M.D. Tina S. Richman, M.D. Edward B. Strauss, M.D.

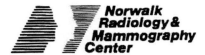

**Norwalk
Radiology &
Mammography
Center**

148 East Avenue, Norwalk, CT 06851
(203) 838-4886

KESAVAN NAIR, M.D.   05/01/89
40 CROSS STREET
NORWALK, CT.   06851

DEAR DR. NAIR:

In reference to your recent referral of:

S. A

05/01/89 08:00   CT HEAD WITH CONTRAST

Examination: CT Scan Head With Contrast

5 mm overlapping sections were obtained from base to vertex
following the infusion of contrast. The study was compared to
the most recent CT exam of ~~1/18/89~~. 3/7/89

Again identified is evidence of metastatic disease involving the
right frontal region, left occipital lobe and right temporal
region. In comparison to the last previous exam, this now
appears to have developed increased edema and increased size in
the overall diameter of the enhancing component of the
intracranial metastases.

The right temporal region demonstrates a 3 cm - 3.5 cm enhancing
component in the anterior middle-cranial fossa with extensive
right temporal lobe edema that extends to the right periatrial
region. The left occipital lesion measures approximately 2 cm -
2.5 cm in diameter (approximately the same as previously noted)
but there is increasing left occipital edema, compared to the
previous exam. The enhancing component of the right frontal
lesion, that is parafalcian in location, now measures 2 cm.
Again, there is increased right frontal edema.

There is no evidence of midline shift or extra-axial fluid
collections. No osseous obstruction is evident.

IMPRESSION:

Increased intracranial edema and size of previously reported
intracranial metastases when compared to ~~1/18/89~~. 3/7/89

Thank you for referring Mr. A   to our office

JAMES BAUMAN, M.D.

James S. Bauman, M.D. William T. Cronin, M.D. Alan H. Levine, M.D. Richard J. Lisi, M.D. Avelino N. Maitem, M.D.
Chris McGarry, M.D. Pradip Pathare, M.D. Alan H. Richman, M.D. Tina S. Richman, M.D. Edward B. Strauss, M.D.

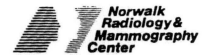

Norwalk Radiology & Mammography Center

148 East Avenue, Norwalk, CT 06851
(203) 838-4886

KESAVAN NAIR, M.D.   07/02/89
40 CROSS STREET
NORWALK, CT.   06851

DEAR DR. NAIR:

In reference to your recent referral of:

S. A

06/30/89 12:00   CT ABDOMEN WITH CONTRAST

Examination: CT of the Abdomen

CT of the abdomen is compared with a previous abdominal CT done
3/8/89.

The current study again shows evidence of a right pneumonectomy.
The liver is without focal abnormalities. The pancreas is
unremarkable.

The left adrenal mass has probably increased minimally since the
last study, currently measuring approximately 2.5 x 3.5 x 5 cm.

No retroperitoneal or other abdominal lymphadenopathy is seen.
The kidneys are without mass or hydronephrosis.

IMPRESSION:

Left adrenal mass has minimally increased in size since the
previous study of 3/8/89. The mass measures approximately 2.5 x
3.5 x 5 cm.

Thank you for referring Mr. A.   to our office

CHRIS MCGARY, M.D.

XCR: ODE/I

James S. Bauman, M.D. William T. Cronin, M.D. Alan H. Levine, M.D. Richard J. Lisi, M.D. Avelino N. Maitem, M.D.
Chris McGary, M.D. Pradip Pathare, M.D. Alan H. Richman, M.D. Tina S. Richman, M.D. Edward B. Strauss, M.D.

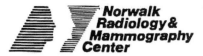

Norwalk Radiology & Mammography Center

148 East Avenue, Norwalk, CT 06851
(203) 838-4886

KESAVAN NAIR, M.D.   07/02/89
40 CROSS STREET
NORWALK, CT. 06851

DEAR DR. NAIR:

In reference to your recent referral of:

S. A

06/30/89-13:00   CT HEAD WITH CONTRAST

Examination: CT of the Head

Comparison is made with a CT of the head of 5/1/89.

The current CT of the head shows decrease in size of the three metastatic lesions present on the previous study. Specifically, the right temporal lobe lesion now measures approximately 1.5 x 2 cm. The left occipital lesion is approximately 1.5 cm in diameter (previously approximately 2 cm). The right frontal dural based lesion measures approximately 1 cm in diameter. There is decreased edema around all three lesions.

No new metastatic lesions are identified in the head.

IMPRESSION:

The three metastatic lesions on the 5/1/89 CT have decreased in size. No new metastatic lesions are seen.

Thank you for referring Mr. A   to our office

CHRIS MCGARY, M.D.

XCR: ODE/I

James S. Bauman, M.D. William T. Cronin, M.D. Alan H. Levine, M.D. Richard J. Lisi, M.D. Avelino N. Maitem, M.D.
Chris McGary, M.D. Pradip Pathare, M.D. Alan H. Richman, M.D. Tina S. Richman, M.D. Edward B. Strauss, M.D.

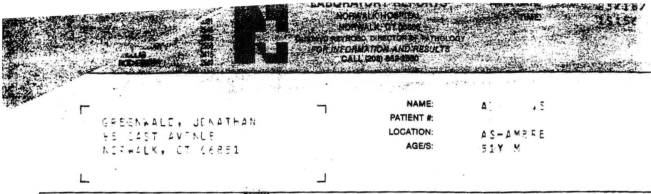

GREENWALD, JONATHAN
45 EAST AVENUE
NORWALK, CT 06851

NAME:	A S
PATIENT #:	
LOCATION:	AS-AMREE
AGE/S:	51Y M

T3316   COLL: 03/16/87 15:30   REC: 03/17/87 08:00 PHYS: GREENWALD, JONATH

FINE NEEDLE ASP.
   SITE   WANG NEEDLE ASPIRATION OF LUNG
   CYTOLOGY NUMBER   C87 2674
   FNA NUMBER   38
   NUMBER OF SLIDES   4
   DIAGNOSIS   POSITIVE FOR MALIGNANT CELLS,
                              ADENOCARCINOMA IN TYPE.
   PATHOLOGIST   SARASWATHI NAIR, MD
   ATTENTION   FOR ADDITIONAL INFORMATION ON THIS
                           SPECIMEN PLEASE SEE CYTOLOGY FINE
                           NEEDLE ASPIRATION REPORT.

END OF REPORT   PAGE 2

THORACIC AND CARDIOVASCULAR ASSOCIATES OF NEW HAVEN, P. C.

CARDIAC, THORACIC AND VASCULAR SURGERY

40 TEMPLE STREET · NEW HAVEN, CONNECTICUT 06510
789-2200

HAROLD STERN, M.D.   RICHARD K SHAW, M.D

ALLAN L. TOOLE, M.D.   WILLIAM C. SCOTT, M.D.

RALPH W. DeNATALE, M.D.   RONALD B. PONN, M.D.

August 5, 1987

Jonathan Greenwald, M.D.
85 East Avenue
Norwalk, Conn. 06851

    Re: S. A

         Admission: 7/28/87 Yale-New Haven Hospital- Service of Dr. Ponn
         Diagnosis: Adenocarcinoma right lung, stage III ($T_1N_2M_0$)
         Operation: 7/29/87 Fiberoptic bronchoscopy, right radical
                     pneumonectomy- Dr. Ponn
         Discharge: 8/5/87 Service of Dr. Ponn

Dear Dr. Greenwald:

Mr. A.   did well postoperatively. His final pathology showed adenocarcinoma
with extensive hilar node involvement and one positive subcarinal mediastinal
node. In view of the latter finding, I have recommended that he undergo adjuvant chemotherapy and radiation therapy for local and distant control. He
has spoken to the oncologist and will consider the matter before making a final
decision.

I will see him back in the office in a couple of weeks for an x-ray and I'll
let you know how things are going and what he has decided.

Sincerely yours,

Ronald B. Ponn, M.D.

RBP:amf

cc: Leonard Farber, M.D., 60 Temple Street, New Haven, Conn. 06510
     Arthur Knowlton, M.D.,Hospital of Saint Raphael, Radiation Therapy Department,
     1450 Chapel Street, New Haven, Conn. 06511

THE NORWALK MEDICAL GROUP, P. C.

40 CROSS STREET

NORWALK, CONNECTICUT 06851

—

AREA CODE: 203 845-2000

INTERNAL MEDICINE
JAMES J. GRIFFITH, M. D.
DENNIS G. HUSKINS, M. D
RICHARD G. HUNTLEY, JR., M. D.

INTERNAL MEDICINE-CARDIOLOGY
JOHN J. SACCO, M. D.
WILLIAM M. SULLIVAN, M. D

ENDOCRINOLOGY
JEROME JOSHUA KLEIN, M. D.

HEMATOLOGY-ONCOLOGY
PAUL L. SCHULMAN, M. D

ONCOLOGY
ANTHONY G. COSCIA, M. D.
KESAV G. NAIR M. D.

GASTROENTEROLOGY
PAUL E. SCHWARTZ, M. D.

INFECTIOUS DISEASES
ERNEST ATLAS, M. D.
ARTHUR YEE, M. D

INFECTIOUS DISEASES-ADULT ALLERGY
MARVIN DEN, M. D.

RENAL DISEASES
PAUL B WIENER, M. D

RHEUMATOLOGY
STUART N NOVACK, M. D

PULMONARY DISEASES
A. JOEL PAPOWITZ, M. D
ANDREW M MURPHY, M. D

RADIOLOGY CONSULTANTS
RADIOLOGY ASSOCIATES OF
WESTPORT, P. C.

March 10, 1989

Jonathan G. Greenwald, M.D.
148 East Avenue
Norwalk, Connecticut

                              Re: . . . .

Dear Jonathan:

   Mr. A   was in the office today for a follow-up. He is feeling a
little better at this time and also stronger. He is currently on 5 mg. of
Prednisone a day. His appetite is reasonably good and his weight has been
stable. He gets headaches very rarely now, and there are no significant
neurologic symptoms. He does have some low back pain but is unchanged from
before.

   On physical examination the blood pressure was 120/70. There was no
lymphadenopathy. The left lung was clear. The abdomen revealed no
hepatomegaly or masses. Neurologic examination revealed no cranial nerve
abnormalities, cerebellar dysfunction or motor dysfunction.

   A CT scan of the abdomen done earlier in the week revealed no change in
the size of the left adrenal mass. A whole body bone scan, which had
previously shown slight increased activity in the sphenoid ridge, is now
normal except for increased activity in the right ankle where he is known to
have had trauma.

   His condition appears to be stable at this time and it is reasonable to
withhold any chemotherapy until there are clear signs for progression. (if any)

                      With best regards,

KGN/mh   Kesav G. Nair, M.D.
cc: Nicholas J. Gonzalez

12. Patient: LE
DOB: 9/26/29

Patient LE is a 63 year-old white male filmmaker with a history of metastatic adenocarcinoma of the lung. He had been in good health until September 1990 when he developed severe chronic headaches while on a trip to India. Upon returning to the U.S. in November 1990, he was hospitalized at New York University for an evaluation. At that time CT of the head revealed a lesion in the right cerebellar hemisphere with edema, mass effect, and mild hydrocephalus. Chest X-ray revealed a left lung lesion, confirmed by CT scan.

Patient LE underwent resection of the brain lesion on November 16, 1990 at NYU. The pathology report describes metastatic papillary adenocarcinoma, moderately differentiated, consistent with a lung primary. After recovering from his brain surgery, patient LE was then admitted to Memorial Sloan-Kettering where on December 13, 1990, the left upper lobe lung tumor was resected. The pathology report describes adenocarcinoma, with 13 nodes negative for cancer. Patient LE subsequently underwent a course of 5500 rads of full brain radiation, completed in early March 1991. He never received chemotherapy.

Patient LE first came to see me on May 2, 1991. At that time, he complained of significant memory loss, balance disturbances, and problems with concentration that he feared would affect his career. His only medication was Procardia, prescribed for mild hypertension. His examination and blood work were unremarkable, except for the described mental status changes.

Since that time, patient LE has followed his nutritional protocol and has done well, with no evidence of recurrent disease. His physicians at NYU and Sloan-Kettering follow him as well as myself. He was last seen by me in June 1993, and was feeling well, with significant improvement in his memory, concentration and intellectual capacities. He is currently working on a book as well as a documentary film.

The median survival from time of diagnosis for patients with adenocarcinoma of the lung with a single brain metastasis, treated with radiation and surgery, runs from 9–18 months, with the best results at Memorial. Patient LE is coming up to three years since his diagnosis, and has completed two years on his nutritional protocol. I present him as an unusual case of long-term survival with poor prognosis cancer, although he has not enjoyed documented regression of existing disease on my therapy.

Dr. Gonzalez presented these 25 cancer case studies to the NCI in 1993 and then updated the patient status information in 2001. Below are Dr. Gonzalez's personal notes with updated survival information:

Metastatic lung cancer to brain. Did very well then quit program, and eventually died 8 years out.

7026 10-79

HG NO. & ACCESSION D

OPERATIVE DIAGNOSIS:

TISSUE SPECIMEN HISTORY   OPERATIVE FINDINGS:

6 yo man with headache of unbalance and cerebellar lesion c/w met on MRI. Lung primary implied since CT chest shows solitary lesion. Impression: metastatic lesion to brain possibly lung.   Doyle

	REF	PAY'T	PHYSICIAN NAME		CODE #	FC-1
	DATE		RECEIPT NO.			AMOUNT

POST OPERATIVE DIAGNOSIS:
S/A

PRIOR OPERATIONS: ☐ NYU Date:	☐ ELSEWHERE	Date:

SURGEON   COPIES TO DR. (S)
Dr. J. Ransohoff   DO NOT WRITE BELOW

FINAL DIAGNOSIS WITH GROSS AND MICROSCOPIC DESCRIPTION:

DIAGNOSIS
Metastatic papillary adenocarcinoma, moderately differentiated

GROSS DESCRIPTION
Specimen received in formalin labelled "cerebellar metastatic mass" consists of a round, soft yellow-tan piece of tissue measuring 1.3 x 1 x 0.4 cm. In toto as "A".

MICROSCOPIC EXAMINATION
A: This shows a necrotic epithelial neoplasm. The tumor cell have round or elongated slightly hyperchromatic or pale nuclei prominent single or multiple nucleoli. The cells have vacuola slightly eosinophilic abundant cytoplasm. These cells formed numrous and distorted glandular and papillary structures. The are numerous often atypical mitotic figures. Focally the tumc abutts on atrophic cerebellar cortex. The tumor has clearly defined margins, however, isolated areas of infiltration are noticed.

RK   J. Lopez, M.D./D. Zagzag, M.D./G.N. Budzilovi
                                              PATHOLOGIST SIGNATUR

SNOMED CODE(S):
T-X6000; M-80503

NO. SLIDES EXAMINED: 1	PATHOLOGY CODE: 1	T.R. CODE: GROSS PICTURE	DATE OF REPORT 11/9/9

1990 NOV -6 PM 9:27

NEW York, N.Y. 1002   1275 YORK AVE., NY, NY 10021
SURGICAL PATHOLOGY

SUBMITTED BY DOCTOR _Martin_

OUTSIDE SOURCE

958503   M   61/P
1   .E
12227153   MARTIN

M-1520B

PATIENT NAME AND ADDRESS

LABORATORY USE ONLY

FSP: LEVEL 11 LEFT MEDIAS   SP: LEVEL 5 LEFT MEDIAST
TINAL L.N.   INAL L.N.
FSP: LEFT UPPER LOBE LUNG   SP: LEVEL 9 LEFT MEDIAST
                             INAL L.N.
SP: L.N. OVER SUP. PULMO
NARY VEIN

ANATOMIC SOURCE OF SPECIMEN _Lg lung_

ACCESSION DATE AND NUMBER

CLINICAL DIAGNOSIS _R/o Carcinoma_

026938 DE 13 90

PREVIOUS ACCESSIONS IN THIS LABORATORY   ☐ YES   ☐ NO   PREVIOUS PATHOLOGY NUMBERS

SIGNIFICANT CLINICAL DATA (USE ANATOMIC STAMPS WHEN POSSIBLE)

AGE _61_   SEX _M_

61 yo ♂ c̄ left lung mass

DISPOSITION OF REPORT IF OTHER THAN CHART

DATE OF REPORT _12/17/90_   **PATHOLOGY REPORT**
(SEE REVERSE SIDE FOR GROSS PATHOLOGY)
P. Lieberman : ch   1/0

<8658

MICROSCOPIC REPORT BY DR. _____

1. FROZEN SECTION: Benign.
    PARAFFIN SECTION: Negative level 11 left mediastinal lymph node.
2. FROZEN SECTION: Benign (bronchial margin).
    PARAFFIN SECTION: Moderately to poorly differentiated
    adenocarcinoma of the apical-posterior segment of left upper lobe of
    lung. Negative bronchial, vascular and pleural margins. Negative
    peribronchial lymph nodes (0/4).
3. Negative superior pulmonary vein lymph nodes (0/5).
4. Negative level 5 left mediastinal lymph nodes (0/2).
5. Negative level 9 left mediastinal lymph node (0/1).

PATH. REPORT
11
P-0965

CHART COPY

DESCRIPTION OF GROSS PATHOLOGY BY DR.   Dr. Fagel/cj   12/13/90

1. CLINICAL DIAGNOSIS: Rule out carcinoma left lung
   SOURCE OF SPECIMEN: Level 11 left mediastinal lymph node
   FROZEN SECTION DIAGNOSIS: Benign

Now in formalin is a portion of anthracotic lymph node measuring 1.5cm
in widest diameter. Entirely submitted.

SUMMARY OF SECTIONS:
FSC - frozen section control 1

                           Dr. Fagel/cj   12/13/90

2. CLINICAL DIAGNOSIS: Rule out carcinoma left lung
   SOURCE OF SPECIMEN: Left upper lobe lung, freeze bronchial
                                margin
   FROZEN SECTION DIAGNOSIS: Benign

Received fresh is the left upper lobe of lung weighing 280g and
measuring 23 x 9 x 3cm in greatest dimension. A subpleural tumor
measuring 3 x 2.5 x 2.5cm is present with pleural puckering in the
apical posterior segment. The tumor is noted 7cm from the bronchial
margin. On sectioning the tumor has a firm tan grayish/yellowish
somewhat mucoid cut surface with circumscribed borders. The bronchial
mucosa is unremarkable. The rest of the lung shows mild anthracotic
changes and congestive cut surfaces.

SUMMARY OF SECTIONS:
FSC - frozen section control   1
P   - primary tumor   3
AB - adjacent bronchial margin 1
VM - vascular margin   4
PL - peribronchial lymph nodes Aggregate
R   - random section   1
TOTAL Multiple

                           Dr. Fagel/cj   12/13/90

3. CLINICAL DIAGNOSIS: Rule out carcinoma left lung
   SOURCE OF SPECIMEN: Lymph node over superior pulmonary vein

Received in formalin are several small irregular fragments of fatty
tissue and portions of anthracotic lymph nodes measuring in aggregate
1.5 x 1 x 0.5cm. Entirely submitted.

SUMMARY OF SECTIONS:
Undesignated Aggregate

                           Dr. Fagel/cj   12/13/90

4. CLINICAL DIAGNOSIS: Rule out carcinoma left lung
   SOURCE OF SPECIMEN: Level 5 left mediastinal lymph node

Received in formalin are 2 portions of partially anthracotic lymph nodes
each measuring approximately 0.6cm in widest diameter. Entirely

11/06/90
06:21 PM

```
                                            NSICU8
   0444184   77297   09/26/29   61   M
   FOO SUN-HOO MD                                                        I    F
```

ORDER: C.T. CHEST   43.01

TRANSCRIBER: PGAL

RADIOLOGIST: MCCAULEY,DOROTHY I.

EXAMINATION PERFORMED: 11/05/90 RESULTS FOR: C.T. CHEST

BEGINNING ABOVE THE STERNAL NOTCH AND EXTENDING DOWN BELOW THE
DIAPRHAGM THE CHEST WAS SCANNED AT 10 MM. INTERVALS WITHOUT
INTRAVENOUS CONTRAST MATERIAL.

THE MEDIASTINAL STRUCTURES ARE NORMAL. THERE IS A MARKED PECTUS
EXCAVATUM DEFORMITY CAUSING COMPRESSION OF THE CARDIAC STRUCTURES.

THE HILAR STRUCTURES ARE NORMAL. THE MAJOR, LOBAR AND SEGMENTAL
BRONCHI ARE PATENT AND NORMAL.

IN THE LUNGS THERE IS AN IRREGULARLY MARGINATED MASS LESION IN THE
LEFT LUNG APEX WHICH MEASURES APPROXIMATELY 2.5 CM. IN DIAMETER. THE
LUNGS ARE OTHERWISE CLEAR.

IMPRESSION: IRREGULAR MASS LESION IN THE LEFT APEX AS DESCRIBED.
MOST PROBABLY REPRESENTS PRIMARY PULMONARY NEOPLASM. NO EVIDENCE OF
ANY MEDIASTINAL OR HILAR ADENOPATHY.

DD/DT 11/6/90 PMG

C.T. CHEST   11/06/90

NEW YORK UNIVERSITY MEDICAL CENTER

L F   NSICU8
0944184   77297   09/26/29   61   M
FOO SUN-HOO MD

L F

ORDER: M.R.I. GENERAL POSTERIOR FOSSA   19.01

TRANSCRIBER: RCAU

RADIOLOGIST: KRICHEFF, IRVIN I.
                 SANCHEZ, GUSTAVO

EXAMINATION PERFORMED: 11/03/90 RESULTS FOR: M.R.I. GENERAL POSTERIOR
FOSSA

AFTER THE ADMINISTRATION OF INTRAVENOUS GD-DTPA, MULTIPLE SAGITTAL T-
1, AXIAL T-1, PROTON DENSITY AND T-2 IMAGES OF THE BRAIN WERE
OBTAINED.

FINDINGS:
THERE IS THE PRESENCE OF A RING ENHANCING LESION IN THE RIGHT
CEREBELLAR HEMISPHERE WITH SURROUNDING EDEMA AND MASS EFFECT GIVEN
BY SLIGHT DISPLACEMENT OF THE FOURTH VENTRICLE AS WELL AS MILD
HYDROCEPHALUS. THE DIFFERENTIAL DIAGNOSIS INCLUDES PRIMARY TUMOR AS
WELL AS METASTATIC DISEASE. NO OTHER AREAS OF ABNORMAL SIGNAL ARE
SEEN WITHIN THE BRAIN PARENCHYMA. THE PITUITARY IS WITHIN NORMAL
LIMITS.

IMPRESSION:
RING ENHANCING LESION WITH EDEMA, MASS EFFECT, AS WELL AS MILD
HYDROCEPHALUS. THE POSSIBILITIES INCLUDE PRIMARY TUMOR VS.
METASTATIC DISEASE.

M.R.I. GENERAL POSTERIOR FOSSA   11/06/90

Lymphoma

13. Patient: MJ
DOB: 5/28/42

Patient MJ is a 52 year-old white woman from Texas with a history of diffuse mixed lymphoma. Patient MJ had previously been in good health when in the fall of 1987 she first developed vague abdominal discomfort. This gradually worsened, and in January of 1988, her physician referred her for an abdominal CT scan that revealed several large abdominal tumors. On January 1, 1989 at Huguley Memorial Medical Center, Fort Worth, Texas, she underwent exploratory surgery, hysterectomy and bilateral salpingo-oophorectomy, and resection of two large 10 cm. masses attached at the mesentery. The pathology report describes diffuse mixed lymphoma, mixed small and large cleaved cell type.

Patient MJ then completed six months of chemotherapy with MACOP-B. Repeat CT scans in August 1988, at the completion of chemotherapy, were negative and she was assumed to be in remission. Subsequent scans were clear until May of 1991 when an abdominal CT picked up two nodules in the lungs, the largest in the lingula measuring 1.6 cm, the smaller in the left lower lobe measuring 0.6 cm. Chest CT on July 23, 1991 revealed a 2.5 by 2 cm. mass in the left hilar area and an abnormality of the lingula in its anterior aspect. A possible left lower lobe mass was also described. CT scan of chest on August 8, 1991, without contrast, demonstrated a vague infiltrate in the lingular segment of the left upper lobe, felt to be scar because of lack of change from CT scan done 3 weeks earlier.

Although chemotherapy was discussed, patient MJ had learned of my work and decided to pursue my program. She was first seen in my office on September 12, 1991 and at that time, she felt well, with no complaints. She was on Premarin 0.625 mg per day. Her examination was unremarkable.

After returning to Texas, patient MJ began her nutritional protocol. After six months on her therapy, a repeat CT scan on March 31, 1992 indicated a small pleural based density associated with the anterior lateral left cardiac margin closely associated with the epicardial fat pad, approximately 1 by 1.5 cm in size, of unclear significance. This represents a significant reduction in size from the prior scans of 1991. Furthermore, the additional lesions documented on the previous studies were not detected. A more recent CT scan of the abdomen was clear.

Patient MJ has now completed nearly two years on her nutritional protocol, and has suffered ups and downs, but she is compliant with her program, and in good health. When I last spoke with her in June 1993, she was well, with no complaints.

Dr. Gonzalez presented these 25 cancer case studies to the NCI in 1993 and then updated the patient status information in 2001. Below are Dr. Gonzalez's personal notes with updated survival information:

Stage IV lymphoma. Alive and well 9 years out. No sign of disease. This patient's survival status was updated again in 2016. Please refer to page 257 for this additional information.

CLINICAL DIAGNOSIS: PATHOLOGY NO.:   S88-121

MACROSCOPIC + MICROSCOPIC EXAMINATION: DATE OF OPERATION: 1-18-88

GROSS DESCRIPTION

A. Labeled "Node (superior mesenteric artery node)
Received is an oval tan mass measuring 1.8 x 1.0 x 0.7 cms. A portion
is submitted for frozen section and the remainder for permanent sectioning.

FROZEN SECTION DIAGNOSIS

POSSIBLE LYMPHOMA.

B. Labeled "Mesenteric mass"
Received are multiple large oval smooth-surfaced red-tan glistening
masses measuring together 9.0 x 8.0 x 8.0 cms. Cut surface throughout
these masses shows smooth tan glistening solid interior. Representative
portions are submitted for both frozen sectioning and multiple sections
for permanent sectioning, including several touch preparations.

FROZEN SECTION DIAGNOSIS

LYMPHOMA, PERMANENTS PENDING.

C. Labeled "Uterus with tubes and ovaries"
Received is a uterus with bilateral tubes and ovaries. The left ovary
is distorted with a cyst filled with clear fluid. It measures overall
4.5 x 4.0 x 3.0 cms. The accompanying fallopian tube is tortuous and
measures 4.0 x 0.7 x 0.6 cms. A representative portion of this cyst
and tube, which is partially adhesed to it, is submitted lettered "L."
The right ovary measures 2.5 cms in greatest dimension and the accompanying
tube measures 5.0 x 0.7 x 0.7 cms. A representative section to include
the ovary and tube is submitted lettered "R." The uterus weighs 170.0
gms and measures 10.5 x 6.5 x 5.0 cms. The cervix is pale and measures
3.0 cms across. The serosa is tan, smooth and glistening. Two sections
from the cervix are submitted. Opening the uterus shows pink-tan velvety
endometrium measuring up to 0.2 cms in thickness. Cut section through
the uterus shows tan smooth stroma and representative sections to include
the endometrium, myometrium, and serosa are are submitted. Cut surface
also includes an occasional gray-white nodular mass with a swirled
pattern on cut surface. The largest of these measures up to 0.6 cms
in greatest dimension and a representative portion is submitted.

D. Labeled "Mesenteric lymph nodes"
Received are two pink-tan soft tissue fragments measuring together
2.5 x 1.4 x 0.5 cms and are submitted in their entirety.

Continued/.....

101

PATIENT IDENTIFICATION:	
NAME:	M. J.
M. R. NO.	AGE 45
HOSPITAL NO.	
ATTENDING PHYSICIAN	Dr L Whitcomb/W Perryman
ROOM NO.	109

PATHOLOGY REPORT
HUGULEY MEMORIAL MEDICAL CENTER
FORT WORTH, TEXAS

Page 2.

CLINICAL DIAGNOSIS: PATHOLOGY NO.:   S88-121

MACROSCOPIC + MICROSCOPIC EXAMINATION: DATE OF OPERATION: 1-18-88

GROSS DESCRIPTION (CONT'D)

E. Labeled "Nevus of skin near xyphoid"
Received is a pale tan skin fragment with a dark gray-black lesion
in its mid portion. The lesion measures less than 0.1 cm across. It
is bisected and submitted in toto.

MICROSCOPIC DESCRIPTION

Multiple permanent and frozen sections lettered A and B show a lymphoma
characterized by a diffuse relatively monotonous sheet of lymphoma
cells. There is a mixture of both small dark relatively mature lymphocytes
with small and large lymphoma cells with a histiocytic type appearance.
Many of these larger cells have multiple micronucleoli with an occasional
larger nucleolus. Mitoses are also occasionally encountered. Some
areas have a slightly more polymorphous infiltrate with some areas
having eosinophils. However, careful searching does not reveal any
Reed-Sternberg cells and the overall histologic features are those
of a diffuse lymphoma of a mixed small and large cleaved cell type.
Several touch preparations are also included in this study.

C. These sections show portions of an ovary with a large simple cyst
and adjacent fallopian tube with multiple mesonephric rests and mild
fibrosis. Sections of the right ovary include a convoluted corpus
luteum and simple cyst. The adjacent portion of fallopian tube shows
fibrosis and mesonephric rests in the serosa. Sections of the cervix
show benign squamous epithelium which is lightly keratinized and overlies
areas of stroma containing multiple Nabothian cysts and an infiltrate
of chronic inflammatory cells. Sections of the endometrium show a
lush secretory endometrium with moderate cellularity and even scattering
of tortuous glands. Other sections include myometrium with portions
of nodular masses composed of interlacing bundles of spindle-shaped
smooth muscle cells.

D. These sections show portions of lymphoid tissue with reactive sinus
histiocytosis and a scattering of germinal centers. There is no evidence
of lymphoma involvement by these lymph nodes.

E. Sections show lightly keratinized skin and underlying tissue. Centrally
there is a scattering of nevus cells along the junction which contain
an abundance of coarse brown pigment. There is no significant cytologic
atypia and these collective features are those of a pigmented junctional
nevus.

Continued/.....

101

PATHOLOGY REPORT
HUGULEY MEMORIAL MEDICAL CENTER
FORT WORTH, TEXAS

PATIENT IDENTIFICATION:

NAME:	M , J
M. R. NO.	AGE 45
HOSPITAL NO.	
ATTENDING PHYSICIAN	Dr L Whitcomb
ROOM NO.	109

Page 3.

CLINICAL DIAGNOSIS: PATHOLOGY NO.:   S88-121

MACROSCOPIC + MICROSCOPIC EXAMINATION: DATE OF OPERATION: 1-18-88

DIAGNOSES

A. TISSUE FROM SUPERIOR MESENTERIC LYMPH NODE AREA: DIFFUSE LYMPHOMA, MIXED SMALL
    AND LARGE CLEAVED CELL TYPE.

B. TISSUE FROM MESENTERIC MASS: DIFFUSE LYMPHOMA, MIXED SMALL AND LARGE CLEAVED
    CELL TYPE.

C. CERVIX: MILD CHRONIC CERVICITIS.
            MULTIPLE NABOTHIAN CYSTS.

    UTERUS: LEIOMYOMA.
             SECRETORY ENDOMETRIUM.

    RIGHT OVARY: CORPUS LUTEUM.
                  SIMPLE CYST.

    LEFT OVARY: LARGE SIMPLE CYST.

    RIGHT AND LEFT FALLOPIAN TUBES: MILD FIBROSIS WITH SEROSAL MESONEPHRIC RESTS.

D. TISSUE FROM MESENTERIC LYMPH NODES: REACTIVE SINUS HISTIOCYTOSIS.

E. TISSUE FROM SKIN: PIGMENTED JUNCTIONAL NEVUS.

DGT:jk

D G Toler, MD

101

D: 1-19-88
T: 1-19-88
Code 7   PATHOLOGY REPORT
     HUGULEY MEMORIAL MEDICAL CENTER
          FORT WORTH, TEXAS

PATIENT IDENTIFICATION:

NAME: M____, J
M. R. NO.   AGE 45
HOSPITAL NO.
ATTENDING PHYSICIAN Dr L Whitcomb
ROOM NO.   109

```
                                    J.
                                       ...
                                    Duncanville, Texas ...
                                     (214) 780-0882
```

Charles Duer, M. D.
900 W. Randol Mill Rd.
Suite 117
Arlington, Texas 76012

                    McCOY,

            11/26/90   27272

EXAMINATION: CT OF THE ABDOMEN AND PELVIS

FINDINGS AND INTERPRETATION: Our examination is reviewed and compared
to an outside study from Hugly Hospital dated 5/5/90. The described
lymphadenopathy in our current study was re-evaluated and felt to be
present in the periaortic area and anterior to the aorta and compared to
the Hugly study in June, 1990 where lymphadenopathy was noted. There
has been no overall significant change since June. The lymphadenopathy
is small with no masses or large lymph nodes identified. No other
changes since the June study were identified.

CONCLUSION: Mild periaortic lower abdominal lymphadenopathy was noted,
unchanged since June, 1990.

Thank you for this referral.

Consultants In Diagnostic Imaging

Victor E. McCall, M. D.
Diplomate American Board of Radiology

VEM:45
d/t: 2/6/91

```
DUNCANVILLE DIAGNOSTIC CENTER          CENTRAL DIAGNOSTIC CENTER
     718 W. Wheatland Road                1310 Stemmons Avenue
   Duncanville, Texas  75137                   Suite 102
                                          Dallas, Texas  75208

       (214) 780-0882                        (214) 941-2711
--------------------------------------------------------------------

Charles Duer, M. D.
801 Road to Six Flags
Suite 106
Arlington, Texas 76012
```

PATIENT NAME: M . . . , J(. . .   AGE: 48 :   42)

DATE OF EXAM: 11/26/90   X-RAY #: 27272

EXAMINATION: CT OF THE ABDOMEN

FINDINGS AND INTERPRETATION: Multiple 8 mm. transaxial views of the
upper abdomen were obtained after the oral ingestion of contrast
media then repeated after the intravenous injection of contrast media
showing the intra-abdominal anatomy well. The liver, spleen, and
pancreas were unremarkable. There is no periaortic lymphadenopathy
noted. The kidneys were normal in appearance, functioning satis-
factorily with no masses seen.

CONCLUSION: Normal upper abdominal CT evaluation with no metastatic
lesions noted. No lymphadenopathy identified.

EXAMINATION: CT EVALUATION OF THE PELVIS

FINDINGS AND INTERPRETATION: Multiple 8 mm. transaxial views of the
intrapelvic anatomy was performed after the oral and intravenous
injection of contrast media. There is increased size in the anterior
mid abdomen just anterior to the aorta in the upper pelvic region
suggesting lymphadenopathy. No large masses were identified. No
pelvic fluid or ascites was apparent. The lower pelvic area appeared
to be unremarkable.

MC. , J
PAGE TWO

CONCLUSION: Upper pelvic region shows increased size of the lymph
nodes in the periaortic area suggesting lymphadenopathy.   No large
masses were noted. No ascites or other significant findings were
identified.

Thank you for this referral.

Consultants In Diagnostic Imaging

Victor E. McCall, M. D.
Radiologist

VEM:45
d/t; 11/26/90
Report not reviewed by
Radiologist after dictation

Duncanville Diagnostic   Central Diagnostic

718 W. WHEATLAND RD.
DUNCANVILLE, TEXAS 75137
(214) 780-0882

1810 STEMMONS AVE., SUITE 102
DALLAS, TEXAS 75208
(214) 941-2711

Charles Duer, M. D.
801 Road to Six Flags
#106
Arlington, Tx 76012

PATIENT NAME: AGE: 48 (5/88/42)

DATE OF STUDY: 5/24/91   X-RAY #:   27272

HISTORY:

EXAMINATION: CT OF THE ABDOMEN

FINDINGS AND INTERPRETATION: 2 cm transaxial views of the lower chest
and upper abdomen were obtained showing the intraabdominal anatomy
well. There is a nodule in the anterior chest on the left measuring 1.6
cm in diameter, probably within the lingula. There is a smaller one
posteriorly on the left lower lobe measuring approximately 8 mm in
diameter. No effusion was noted. The liver, spleen, and pancreas were
unremarkable. Both kidneys were functioning normally and were
unremarkable. There may be periaortic lymphadenopathy about the aorta
at the level of the kidneys. In review of the prior study, the clinical
lymphadenopathy may have been there previously. If so, it is unchanged
on the current examination.

CONCLUSION: The nodules in the left chest probably in the
            lingula CT of the chest recommended for further
            evaluation.
            Small periaortic lymphadenopathy at the level of the
            kidneys, possibly unchanged from previously seen.
            No other abnormalities seen or altered.

EXAMINATION: CT OF THE PELVIS

FINDINGS AND INTERPRETATION: Multiple transaxial views of the
intrapelvic structures were obtained showing the intrapelvic anatomy
well. The examination is being compared to the previous study of
11/26/90. There has been no overall significant change since the
previous exam. There is a small node with the lymphadenopathy in the
periaortic region. No masses, ascites, or other significant findings
were noted.

RADIOLOGY REPORT

Duncanville Diagnostic

718 W. WHEATLAND RD.
DUNCANVILLE, TEXAS 75137
(214) 780-0882

Central Diagnostic

1010 STEMMONS AVE., SUITE 102
DALLAS, TEXAS 75208
(214) 941-2711

PATIENT NAME: AGE:

DATE OF STUDY: X-RAY:

PAGE TWO

CONCLUSION: A)   Partially visualized
                       previous study.
                B)   No lesion or metastasis

Thank you for this referral.

Consultants in Diagnostic Imaging

Victor M. McNally, M.D.
Diplomate, American Board of Radiology

VEM:
d/t: 5/24/

Duncanville Diagnostic   # *Central Diagnostic*

718 W. WHEATLAND RD.
DUNCANVILLE, TEXAS 75137
(214) 780-0882

1310 STEMMONS AVE., SUITE 102
DALLAS, TEXAS 75208
(214) 941-2711

Charles Duer, M. D.
801 Road to Six Flags
#106
Arlington, Tx 76012

PATIENT NAME: M‍‍, J   AGE: 49   (‍‍‍/42)

DATE OF STUDY: 7/23/91   X-RAY #:

HISTORY:

EXAMINATION: CT OF THE CHEST

FINDINGS AND INTERPRETATION: Multiple 8 mm. transaxial views of the
lower cervical area and intra-thoracic region including a portion of the
upper abdomen were obtained at 8 mm intervals after the oral ingestion
and intravenous injection of contrast media. The lower cervical area
was intact with no masses seen. There was a 2.5 X 2 cm mass in the left
hilar area seen best on cut 189. There is an infiltrate and/or consolidation of the lingula in its anterior aspect. A portion of this
area of density may represent a mass. No old chest CT was available, but
an old abdominal CT was present and the lower lobe was included on that
study where the mass was noted on the study in May 1991. A similar study
obtained in 11/90 did not show this abnormality. Involvement appears to
have increased since the previous study. The right lung remains clear.
No effusion was noted. There may be a second nodule in the posterior
portion of the left lower lobe. The portion of the liver, spleen, and
pancreas visualized was normal. Both kidneys appears to be functioning
and were unremarkable.

CONCLUSION: 1)   Left hilar mass and posterior left lower lobe nodule.
              2)   Progressing mass and associated atelectasis or
                   infiltrate in the lingula.
              3)   No other significant findings were identified on this
                   study.

Thank you for this referral.

Consultants In Diagnostic Imaging

Victor E. McCall, M. D.
Diplomate American Board of Radiology

VEM:

RADIOLOGY REPORT

Methodist
HOSPITALS of DALLAS

DEPARTMENT OF RADIOLOGY
RADIOLOGY REPORT

CHARLTON METHODIST HOSPITAL

NAME: M.   J(
AGE: 49   D.O.B.   -42
REFERRING DR. SWEATT/DEUR/WHITE
ROOM: OP
MED. REC. 208-92-84-0

EXAMINATIONS: CT SCAN OF CHEST
DATE: 8-15-91

CLINICAL INFORMATION: Mass in chest.

Ten mm. thick contiguous axial images were obtained throughout the patient's chest without intravenous contrast. I do not feel intravenous contrast was necessary, as previous CT scan was available for comparison from 3 weeks earlier, which was done with contrast. There is some vague infiltrate in the lingular segment of the left upper lobe, which shows no interval change from the CT scan done 3 weeks ago. Because it has not changed, I suspect it represents some scar tissue from previous infection or trauma. I do not believe it represents a mass lesion or it could represent tumor. I see no mediastinal or hilar or axillary adenopathy. There are no other peripheral lung nodules.

IMPRESSION:

1.   Vague infiltrate in the lingular segment of the left upper lobe whose etiology is likely scarring from old disease. I see no other abnormalities throughout the patient's chest.

FRED BEALL, M.D., D.A.B.R./jah
8-15-91

Proof of Concept

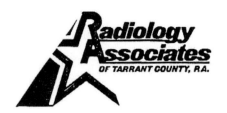

**PENNSYLVANIA AVENUE
IMAGING CENTER**
815 Pennsylvania Avenue
Fort Worth, Texas 76104
Ph:(817)336-8673   Fax:(817)336-1232

```
Pt:   M    J         49y/o      /42)
Dr:   JOHN A JOHNSON, MD      817 645 3930
No:   86830                              Date:  03/31/92

CC:   DR. CHARLES DEUR

86830                                           3/31/92
```

CT SCAN OF THE THORAX:
Axial 10mm interval images were obtained through the thorax after intravenous administration of 100cc Isovue 300 contrast without complication.

There is very slight soft tissue density seen in the area of the thymus in the anterior superior mediastinum not thought to be clinically significant. No indication of mediastinal or hilar adenopathy can be identified. There is a small pleural based density associated with the anterior lateral left cardiac margin closely associated with the epicardial fat pad. This is approximately 1 X 1.5cm in size and is of indeterminate significance. This could merely represent small area of fibrosis. The patient does give a history, however, of a previous abnormal chest x-ray in this region. There is no previous CT for comparison. The remainder of the thorax on CT exam is unremarkable.

IMPRESSION:
THE PATIENT DOES HAVE A SMALL, TRIANGULAR, APPROXIMATELY 1.5CM DENSITY, PLEURAL BASED, ASSOCIATED WITH THE EPICARDIAL FAT PAD ON THE LEFT IN THE MID TO LOWER LUNG FIELD OF INDETERMINATE SIGNIFICANCE.

ROBERT E. GLOYNA, M.D.
11:39AM/wer
C/3:26/wer

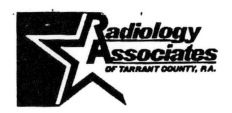

PENNSYLVANIA AVENUE
IMAGING CENTER
815 Pennsylvania Avenue
Fort Worth, Texas 76104
Ph:(817)336-8673   Fax:(817)336-1232

Pt: M\ _ , J.   ᴿ 49y/o   _ _/42)
Dr: JOHN A JOHNSON, MD   817 645 3930
No: 86830   Date: 03/31/92

CC: DR. CHARLES DEUR

86830   _   3/31/92

CT SCAN OF THE ABDOMEN WITH AND WITHOUT CONTRAST:
10mm interval axial images were obtained through the liver before the CT
thoracic study.   Following thoracic CT study, 10mm interval axial images
were extended through the abdomen.   There are small nodes seen in the
paraaortic area, particularly on image #34 through 36. These measure only
1cm in diameter and, therefore, are of questionable significance. This may
well represent normal minimal prominence of the nodes. No significant
adenopathy can be identified. No abdominal mass is noted.

IMPRESSION:
THERE ARE SLIGHTLY PROMINENT NODES ON THE PARA-AORTIC AREA MEASURING UP TO
1CM IN DIAMETER. ABDOMINAL CT, OTHERWISE, IS UNREMARKABLE.

ROBERT E. GLOYNA, M.D.
11:44AM/wer
c/3:26/wer

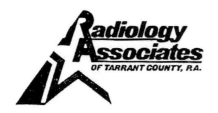

PENNSYLVANIA AVENUE IMAGING CENTER
815 Pennsylvania Avenue
Fort Worth, Texas 76104
Ph:(817)336-8673   Fax:(817)336-1232

Pt: M.   , J   ꓹ 49y/o   ꓷ/42)
Dr: JOHN A JOHNSON, MD   817 645 3930
No: 86830   Date: 03/31/92

CC: DR. CHARLES DEUR

3C·   3/31/92

CT SCAN OF THE PELVIS:
Axial 10mm interval images were obtained through the pelvis following CT
abdominal study and demonstrate no indication of pelvic mass or adenopathy
identified. The appearance would suggest that the patient has had a previous
hysterectomy.

IMPRESSION:
UNREMARKABLE CT PELVIS.

ROBERT E. GLOYNA, M.D.
11:46AM/wer

14. Patient MR
DOB: 1/10/20

Patient MR is a 73 year-old white female from Wisconsin with a history of breast cancer diagnosed in 1957, treated with radical mastectomy and radiation. Patient MR subsequently did well until 1976, when she developed several enlarged bilateral cervical lymph nodes. Her local physician referred her to the Mayo Clinic where biopsies of the nodes revealed malignant lymphoma, diffuse (partially nodular) mixed lymphocytic histiocytic type. Xrays of the chest and a bone survey showed no sign of metastatic disease. However, a bipedal lymphangiogram confirmed suspicious nodes in the region of the lumbar spine, and a bone marrow biopsy was positive for invasive cancer. Overall, the findings indicated advanced lymphoma, as described in the official Mayo summary: "On the basis of the lymphangiogram and the histiologic pattern of the lymphoma, we felt that Patient MR most likely had disseminated disease."

Initially no therapy was advised, but when the neck tumors rapidly grew, Patient MR returned to Mayo in January of 1977 for palliative radiation. She completed a course of radiation therapy to the left supraclavicular, left axillary and mediastinal region. The area of the vertebral column that had been positive on the lymphangiogram was not treated. After Patient MR completed radiation, the Mayo doctors then recommended a course of intensive chemotherapy. However, she refused chemotherapy and instead, after returning home, decided to investigate unconventional cancer therapies. Within weeks, she learned of Dr. Kelley, visited him, and in late January 1977, began the full Kelley program.

Over a five-month period, Patient MR's symptoms improved, and the lymphoma went into remission. At a followup visit to Mayo in May of 1979, she was believed, as reported in her doctor's summary, to be "free of disease."

Patient MR followed her nutritional program for many years, but in the mid-1980's she gradually went off her protocol. In January 1990 she noticed a nodular lesion on her uvula. When this did not resolve, Patient MR went back to Mayo and on March 7, 1990, a 1 cm. uvula nodule was resected. The pathology report documents recurrent nodular lymphoma (low grade). CT of the chest and abdomen, as well as a bone marrow biopsy, were all negative. She was not advised to pursue therapy at that time.

Patient MR first came to my office on March 20, 1990. She reported some fatigue at that time but otherwise was asymptomatic. She was on no medications, and her physical examination was unremarkable.

Patient MR has been my patient now for three years, and overall has followed the Kelley regimen for 17 years. Currently, she remains very compliant with her treatment, is in excellent health and appears disease free. She is followed by her doctors at the Mayo Clinic who have been very pleased with her progress.

Clearly, Patient MR is an unusual patient, now seventeen years out from her diagnosis of diffuse mixed lymphoma.

Dr. Gonzalez presented these 25 cancer case studies to the NCI in 1993 and then updated the patient status information in 2001. Below are Dr. Gonzalez's personal notes with updated survival information:

Stage IV lymphoma. An old Dr. Kelley patient who had a recurrence and began with me in 1990. Survived another 8 years, before dying at age 80.

October 13, 1976

3-231-507

Bernard Street, M.D.
208 South Division Street
Northfield, MN 55057

Dear Doctor Street:

    Mrs. M   R   was recently evaluated in the Lymphoma
Clinic. She had originally been evaluated by Dr. Stephen Cullinan
in the Department of Oncology. Enlarged left supraclavicular lymph
nodes were noted. Biopsy of the left supraclavicular lymph nodes
on October 6, 1976, revealed malignant lymphoma, diffuse (partially
nodular) mixed lymphocytic-histiocytic type. When seen in the Lymphoma
Clinic, there was no sign of residual mass in the left supraclavicular
region and no other sign of active lymphoma on physical examination.

    Chest x-ray was negative. Metastatic bone survey showed no
definite sign of malignancy. Excretory urogram was normal. Bipedal
lymphangiogram revealed suspicious lymph nodes in the region of the
L-2 interspace. Chemistry profile was entirely satisfactory. White
blood count was 5500; hemoglobin, 13.6; platelets, 314,000. Bone
marrow aspiration revealed several focal aggregates of lymphocytes.
suggesting marrow involvement by lymphoma. Bone marrow biopsy, however,
was interpreted as showing no definite evidence of malignant lymphoma.

    On the basis of the lymphangiogram and the histologic pattern
of the lymphoma, we felt that Mrs.   most likely had disseminated
disease. Because she is asymptomatic and has no sign of impending
complications from her lymphoma, we have not advised initiation of
specific therapy at this time.

    We have arranged for a complete re-evaluation in approximately
six weeks. We do intend to initiate treatment at the first sign of
symptomatic progression of her disease.

    Please let us know if we could be of assistance with her case
prior to her scheduled return.

                              Sincerely,

                              M. J. O'Connell, M.D.

MAYO CLINIC
ROCHESTER. MINNESOTA

March 13, 1990

3-231-507

Charles W. Docter, M.D.
Plum City, WI 54761

Dear Doctor Docter:

I am writing you regarding Mrs. M   R   who was at the Mayo
Clinic from March 2-9, 1990. She was initially seen by my colleague,
Dr. Douglas Green in Ear, Nose and Throat, because of a lesion she had
recently discovered in the uvula of her pharynx. As you will recall, she
had a low-grade non-Hodgkin's lymphoma in 1976 which was treated with
radiation therapy here. She has been without evidence of disease ever
since. She has never received any chemotherapy.

On 3-7-90 Doctor Green, under anesthesia, examined the area and found
a 1 cm mass at the free edge of the right faucial arch. This was excised
and found to be a nodular-mixed lymphoma (low-grade). She was referred to
us in Lymphoma Clinic and we saw her on 3-8-90. She has been feeling well
otherwise with no 'B' symptoms and a normal performance status.

Physical examination revealed her to have no peripheral
lymphadenopathy. There was erythema of the right soft palate from the
recent surgery. There was no hepatosplenomegaly.

We staged her with a CT scan of the chest and abdomen which was
negative for adenopathy. The scan showed bilateral peripelvic renal cysts
and a tiny calcified gallstone. Hemoglobin was 13.8 g/dL, white count was
4,700, and platelets were 290,000. Complete blood chemistries were within
normal limits except for a mild increase in her creatinine to 1.1
(0.6-0.9). Other laboratories revealed her to have a normal total
thyroxine, cholesterol 298, and triglycerides 115. Urinalysis was negative
for sugar and protein and microscopic examination was also negative. Urine
culture was negative. The electrocardiogram showed normal sinus rhythm
with a rate of 77 and evidence of a previous anterior infarct, age
undetermined. There was also a non-specific T-wave abnormality. These
changes were not any different than when found on her EKG here in July
1983. Mammogram of the left breast was negative for malignancy. Chest
x-ray showed evidence of a right mastectomy and some fibrosis in the right
base, but was otherwise negative. Bone marrow aspiration and biopsy were
negative.

MAYO CLINIC
ROCHESTER, MINNESOTA

Charles W. Docter, M.D.   -2-   March 13, 1990
3-

She was seen by Dr. James Martenson of Radiation Therapy to get his opinion on whether radiation could be given to the palate area as adjuvant therapy. He pulled her port films from 1976 and it appears that she has received radiation to this area. Therefore, some radiation therapy but not a complete treatment could be administered safely now. We had a long discussion with Mrs. R___. At this time, we have no gross evidence of disease because it has all been excised and the scans and marrow were negative. Because of her long disease-free interval and the still low-grade nature of the lesion that was excised, we felt that a period of observation would also be a reasonable approach as opposed to radiating now. Since only a limited amount of radiation can be given, it may be best to wait and give it at a time when we are sure that there is disease present. I am also reluctant to give her chemotherapy at this time without any evidence of measurable or evaluable disease. Therefore, after discussing this at length with Mr. and Mrs. R___, they are also in agreement to closely observe her. We plan on having her back in two months at which time she will get a re-examination of the palate area.

It certainly was a pleasure seeing Mrs. R___. If you have any questions regarding her evaluation here, please feel free to contact me.

Sincerely yours,

Thomas E. Witzig, M.D.

TEW:cjm
cc: Mrs. M___ R___

MAYO CLINIC
ROCHESTER, MINNESOTA

August 29, 1990

3-231-507

Charles W. Docter, M.D.
Plum City, WI 54761

Dear Doctor Docter:

Mrs. M.   R.   returned on August 24, 1990 in followup for her
low grade lymphoma of the palate. She has been feeling well without any
chemotherapy. She is using enzyme treatment and dietary therapy and feels
good on that.

Physical examination revealed her to have a blood pressure of 140/80,
a pulse of 110, and a weight of 142 pounds. There was no peripheral
lymphadenopathy. Careful examination of her mouth and pharynx revealed no
evidence of recurrence of the lymphoma in the right soft palate area.

Laboratory evaluation revealed a hemoglobin of 13.2 g/dL, a white
count of 4,300 with 71% granulocytes, and a platelet count of 194,000.
Complete blood chemistries were within normal limits except for a slight
elevation of her creatinine to 1.2 (0.6-0.9).

We certainly are very pleased with the way Mrs. R.   is doing and
there is no evidence of any recurrence. She plans on returning here in
three months for followup.

Sincerely yours,

Thomas E. Witzig, M.D.

TEW:cjs
cc: Mrs. M   R

Melanoma

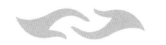

15. Patient KG
11/1/38

Patient KG is a 54 year-old white male with a history of melanoma as well as multiple basal and squamous cell skin cancers. Patient KG is a fair haired and light skinned man who had extensive sun exposure for many years. In 1987 he was first diagnosed with multiple basal and squamous cell skin lesions requiring multiple resections. Then, on September 28, 1988, a lesion above his left ear was biopsied and found to be malignant melanoma, measuring at least 1.3 mm in depth. At that time, a number of cervical nodes were sampled but were clear of cancer.

In the fall of 1988, Patient KG noted a new lesion anterior to his left ear. On August 10, 1989 at Doctor's Hospital in New York he underwent a left superficial parotidectomy and left radical neck dissection. Pathology demonstrated metastatic melanoma to an intraparotid gland lymph node, but with no metastatic disease in the cervical chain. A CT scan of the head, chest and abdomen were all unremarkable.

Patient KG refused all standard therapy for his disease, and instead decided to pursue my therapy. He was first seen in my office on November 9, 1989, and at the time reported a new lesion on the right side of his neck, but otherwise had no complaints. His examination was notable for a 0.5 cm hard nontender node in the right occipital area.

Patient KG proved to be a determined, compliant patient, and has now completed 3.7 years on his nutritional protocol. He is in excellent general health, shows no sign of melanoma, and the dozens of basal and squamous lesions that had been an ongoing problem have gradually resolved.

Dr. Gonzalez presented these 25 cancer case studies to the NCI in 1993 and then updated the patient status information in 2001. Below are Dr. Gonzalez's personal notes with updated survival information:

Metastatic melanoma. Alive and well 11 years out. This patient's survival status was updated again in 2016. Please refer to page 257 for this additional information.

DERM PATH, INC
P.O. BOX 1050
SCARSDALE, N.Y. 10583
(914) 472-0580, (212) 239-0794

PATIENT

PATH. NO. 88-31965-0

SEX   F

DOCTOR: R J FRIEDMAN   MD PC

PECIMEN   LT EAR - A

DATE: 9/28/88   RECVD- 9/19/8

GROSS-   SHAVE 5 X 5 X 3 MM

CLINICAL IMPRESSION-   BCC

MICROSCOPIC DESCRIPTION-   THIS SOMEWHAT PAPULO-NODULAR
MELANOCYTIC NEOPLASM IS CHARACTERIZED BY A FOCALLY INCREASED
NUMBER OF ATYPICAL MELANOCYTES ARRANGED IN CONFLUENT NESTS
ALONG THE DERMO-EPIDERMAL JUNCTION AND SLIGHTLY ABOVE IT.
WITHIN THE DERMIS THERE ARE NESTS AND SHEETS OF ATYPICAL
MELANOCYTES WHICH EXTEND TO THE BASE OF THE SPECIMEN.   THESE
CELLS HAVE PLEOMORPHIC AND HYPERCHROMATIC NUCLEI.   NUMEROUS
ATYPICAL MOTISES ARE PRESENT - 3/HPF.

DIAGNOSIS- MALIGNANT MELANOMA, NEAR LEFT EAR, MEASURING AT LEAST
1.3 MM IN GREATEST THICKNESS
NOTE - WE FAVOR A DIAGNOSIS OF A PRIMARY AMELANOTIC MALIGNANT
MELANOMA.

_____ Edward Heilman, M.D.   Elaine Waldo, M.D.   Craig Austin, M.D.

1ST TUMOR

REMOVED 9/88

DOCTORS HOSPITAL

SURGICAL PATHOLOGY REPORT

90795   Ñ   50
F   SUR
8 10 69   963298 Ps

ECIMEN:	☐ TISSUE	☐ FLUID FOR TUMOR CELLS	☐ OTHER (SPECIFY)	

'ERATING SURGEON.	DATE:	

E-OP AGNOSIS	*Metastatic Melanoma*	LAB. USE ONLY
)ST-OP AGNOSIS		DATE OF SURGERY 8/10/89
JRGICAL OCEDURE	*Parotidectomy + radical neck*	DATE REC'D. 8/11/89
	Dissection	PATH. NO. S-89-5004

ATURE OF SPECIMEN:

2ND TUMOR

LINICAL ATA: REMOVED 8/89

ROZEN SECTION DIAGNOSIS:

PATHOLOGICAL REPORT

:ROSS DESCRIPTION:

The first specimen is submitted as parotid gland, portion and consists of a portion of salivary gland tissue measuring 3.3 x 2.6 x 1.3 cm. At one portion of the tissue part of a grey-white tumor mass is identified. The tumor measures 2 cm in greatest dimensions and appears to be part of a larger tumor mass. NOTE: Rest of the tumor tissue was frozen sectioned for outside special studies. Entire tumor and representative sections of the tissue submitted.

The second specimen is submitted as parotid gland and consists of a portion of salivary gland tissue measuring 2.5 x 1.2 cm in its greatest dimensions. Entire specimen submitted.

The third specimen is submitted as neck content and consists of a radical neck dissection specimen measuring 9 x 5 x 3 cm. It is comprised of the submandibular gland identified with marker #1, skeletal muscle bundles, fibrofatty tissue with lymph nodes and blood vessels. Multiple lymph nodes ranging in size from 0.5 to 1 cm are found embedded within. None of the nodes show gross metastatic tumor. All the lymph nodes are submitted and labelled B to D - posterior triangle. E to G - lower jugular chain and H - upper jugular chain. A is submandibular gland.

RP:sp

MICROSCOPIC DIAGNOSIS:

Metastatic malignant melanoma to intraparotid gland lymph node.

Mild, Chronic inflammation, parotid and submandibular glands.

Reactive hyperplasia, 7 posterior, 12 lower jugular and 5 upper jugular chain lymph
  nodes. No metastatic tumor.

RP:sp

8.15.89	Romulo Prudente, MD
DATE REPORTED	PATHOLOGIST

CPT: 88305
        88304,   88309

Proof of Concept

DOCTORS HOSPITAL | 2ND OPERATION | REPORT OF OPERATION

| K G | MEDICAL RECORD NUMBER | AGE | ROOM | DATE OF SURGERY 8/10/89 |

| SURGEON DR. GOLOMB | 1ST ASSISTANT | DATE OF DICTATION 8/10/89 |

PRE-OP DIAGNOSIS
METASTATIC MELANOMA LEFT PAROTID GLAND.

POST-OP DIAGNOSIS
SAME.

OPERATION PERFORMED
LEFT SUPERFICIAL PAROTIDECTOMY AND LEFT RADICAL NECK DISSECTION
IN CONTINUITY.

ANAESTHESIOLOGIST —   ANAESTHESIA —

FINDINGS:
In the substance of the superficial lobe of the left parotid gland is a 2½ cm diameter mass. This has been previously biopsied by fine needle aspiration and found to contain metastatic melanoma from the primary, which had been on the patient's scalp. The lymph nodes in the neck did not appear to be enlarged or pigmented.

PROCEDURE:
The patient was placed supine on the Operating Room table. The side of the head from the midline anteriorly to the midline posteriorly was prepped with Betadine and included the neck and upper anterior chest. All of this was draped into the field. With a marking pen the planned incisions were drawn on the skin starting in the scalp above the prior scar and running anterior to the ear then curving posteriorly below the tragus and swinging anteriorly along the natural folds of the neck and terminating in the midline anteriorly at the level of the hyoid bone.

The second incision was parallel to the clavicle and 5 cm above it, running from the midline anteriorly to the hairline posteriorly. The skin of these proposed incisions was infiltrated with ½% Lidocaine with epinephrine. The incisions were made and skin flaps were developed superficial to the platysma which was taken with the specimen. The flap on the cheek was extended anteriorly at the level of the roots of the hair follicles to the level of the zygoma arch and over the mandible close to the lateral commissure of the mouth.

Flaps were developed posteriorly to the external auditory cartilage and over the mastoid attachment of the sternocleidomastoid muscle and trapezius muscles. Anteriorly the flaps continued to the midline and inferiorly over the clavicle. The dissection started superiorly by taking all of the tissue down to the skull superiorly and then working anterior to the parotid gland.

Using the Shaw scalpel and the operating telescope, it was possible to identify the branches of the facial nerve going to the eye, forehead and mouth. A nerve stimulator was used to substantiate this observation.

SURGEON COPY

138

REPORT OF OPERATION

DOCTORS HOSPITAL

NAME		MEDICAL RECORD NUMBER	AGE	ROOM	DATE OF SURGERY
K., G.					/ /

SURGEON	1 ST ASSISTANT	DATE OF DICTATION
DR. GOLOMB		8/10/89

PRE-OP DIAGNOSIS

POST-OP DIAGNOSIS

OPERATION PERFORMED

ANAESTHESIOLOGIST —	ANAESTHESIA —

- 2 -

The dissection proceeded posteriorly taking the parotid gland off of the branches of the facial nerve and all of the gland laying superior to the nerve was taken and all of it superficial to the nerve inferior to the ophthalmic branch was taken in the dissection.

The superficial temporal artery and vein were doubly ligated and included in the specimen. The posterior facial vein was doubly ligated and also included. The specimen of the parotid gland was submitted as a complete unit. Part of it was submitted for freezing to be later used in a NCI immunotherapy protocol. The rest of the specimen and the separate portion, which was the lower lobe of the parotid gland, was submitted to Pathology.

The neck dissection then proceeded by dividing the platysma at the level of the margin of the mandible. The marginal mandibular branch of the facial nerve was visualized and spared though it's origins in the parotid gland may have been taken with the lower pole. The submandibular gland was then dissected in it's entirety from beneath the mandible in continuity with the rest of the neck dissection.

Anteriorly the platysma was split along the midline and the dissection then proceeded posteriorly taking the specimen off of the omohyoid and strap muscles. The sternocleidomastoid muscle was divided at the lower end 2 cm above the superior border of the clavicle. The posterior triangle was dissected cleanly off ov the scalene muscles and from beneath the reflection of the trapezius muscle.

The spinal accessory nerve was taken with the specimen. The dissection then proceeded in a cephalad direction taking all of the structures which lay behind, anterior to and superficial to the internal jugular vein. The descendens hypoglossi and ansa hypoglossi nerves were preserved as was the phrenic nerve and the branches of the brachial plexus.

DOCTORS HOSPITAL

REPORT OF OPERATION

NAME		MEDICAL RECORD NUMBER	AGE	ROOM	DATE OF SURGERY
G					/ /

SURGEON	1ST ASSISTANT	DATE OF DICTATION
DR. GOLOMB		8/10/89

PRE-OP DIAGNOSIS

POST-OP DIAGNOSIS

OPERATION PERFORMED

ANAESTHESIOLOGIST —   ANAESTHESIA —

- 3 -

As the dissection proceeded in a cephalad direction it joined
the upper dissection which then proceeded posteriorly, taking
the specimen off the upper end of the jugular vein and in continuity
with the upper portion of the sternocleidomastoid muscle, which
was divided at the mastoid process. The spinal accessory nerve
was divided superiorly and the dissection was then removed from
the upper portion of the posterior triangle.

Markers were placed at the upper end of the jugular chain with
two silk sutures and marker #1 was placed on the submaxillary
gland, marker #2 placed on the posterior triangle and marker
#3 at the lower end of the jugular chain. Hemostasis throughout
was with silk ligatures and the judicious use of electrocoagulation
and the Shaw scalpel.

Estimated blood loss was approximately 100-150 cc. The wound
was thoroughly irrigated with saline at the completion of the
procedure. Two Jackson-Pratt drains were placed in the defect
and sutured to the skin with 00 silk sutures. The incisions
were closed with interrupted subcuticular sutures of 4-0 Vicryl
and the skin was approximated with running subcuticular sutures
of 4-0 prolene supplemented with Steri-Strips. A dry sterile
dressing and Elastoplast tape were applied and patient was sent
to the Recovery Room in good condition.

G/cmn/RR
c.106
8/10/89
8/14/89

DICTATED BY:_____
F. GOLOMB,M.D.

COPY

16. Patient MW
DOB: 11-18-31

Patient MW is a 61 year-old white male research scientist with a history of metastatic melanoma. Patient MW had been in good health when in the spring of 1983, he developed sinus congestion. Over a period of a year, he was treated with a variety of medications without improvement. Eventually, on September 26, 1984, Patient MW underwent nasoseptal reconstruction with resection of two polyps. Pathology evaluation revealed malignant melanoma. Then on November 30, 1984, at Memorial Sloan-Kettering, Patient MW returned to surgery for a left medial maxillectomy, with wide resection of the cribriform plate, both ethmoids, frontal sinus, mucosa of the sphenoid sinuses, resection of the contents of the left maxillary antrum. The nasal septum and right superior turbinate were removed en bloc. The pathology report documents residual disease, but apparently clean margins.

Patient MW received no additional therapy and he did well until late 1986, when routine blood chemistries showed an elevated LDH. No diagnostic investigation was pursued at that point. But in the late spring of 1987, he developed abdominal symptoms including pain, bloating and indigestion. He returned to Memorial for a full metastatic workup: a biopsy of the ethmoid sinus was negative, as was a CT scan of the head. However, an abdominal CT on July 23, 1987 demonstrated a large abdominal mass in the midline extending to the anterior abdominal wall below the level of the umbilicus. On September 14, 1987, he underwent exploratory laparotomy by Alan Turnbull, M.D. at Memorial Hospital and was found to have massive adenopathy in the distal small bowel mesentery invading several loops of small bowel, with tumor seeding in the pelvis adjacent to the main mass. The tumor area itself had ruptured, forming a contained cavity of necrotic tumor adjacent to the terminal ileum. Involved small bowel was resected with primary anastomosis and the tumor was debulked, leaving the capsule of the tumor against the sigmoid colon, base of mesentery, and posterior wall of the bladder. Pathology studies confirmed malignant melanoma.

Patient MW's surgeon told him his disease would prove terminal, and recommended neither chemotherapy nor radiation. However, he decided to pursue nutritional therapy from Robert Atkins, M.D., in New York. Initially, he did well: a CT scan in January 1988—after several months of treatment—was negative. But a follow-up CT scan on May 16, 1988 revealed a soft tissue mass measuring 4.5 × 3.5 cm at the aortic bifurcation compatible with recurrent melanoma. Patient MW returned to his surgeon, who said surgery was inappropriate, and told him he might have six months to live.

Patient MW learned of my work, and initially came to see me on May 28, 1988. At that time, he felt well, and was on no medications. Examination was notable for deviation of the left eye nasally, obvious inguinal adenopathy and a hard mid-pelvic mass. He began his nutritional protocol in June of 1988 and was followed with serial CT scans by his local oncologist in Delaware. A baseline abdominal CT scan on July 12, 1988—shortly after I first met him—documented slight enlargement of the mass (5 by 3.5 cm.) associated with left retroperitoneal and left lower mesenteric adenopathy. Subsequently, there was some slight growth in the main pelvic mass, followed by stabilization and cystification of the tumor over a period of two years. A CT scan on September 7, 1988 showed slight increase in the size of the tumor (4 by 5 cm.) but with improvement in the adenopathy. CT scan on December 22, 1988—six months after Patient MW began his protocol—showed "stable size of mass since CT of 9/7/88 (4.5 by 6 cm.) with resolution of previously described adenopathy." CT scan on June 6, 1989 reported "mass unchanged since 12/22/88…" Then, an MRI in June 1990 revealed that the previously solid mass had evolved into a cystic lesion.

Patient MW remained extremely compliant with his nutritional therapy for over four years, and during this time he enjoyed excellent health. He worked full time, and was asymptomatic. However, in the fall of 1992, he became completely non-compliant with his diet for a number of reasons, and in late fall his local oncologist felt, on physical exam, that the pelvic mass had grown for the first time in years. An abdominal CT scan on December 31, 1992 showed a 7.0 cm soft tissue mass in left mid to lower pelvis, containing areas of necrosis and calcification. A second possible small mass 2.0 cm. and containing calcification was also noted in the right abdomen anterior to the inferior vena cava at the umbilical level.

After discussions with me, Patient MW decided to go to surgery at Memorial for excision of the mass. Preoperative evaluation included CT of the head and abdomen, both negative for metastatic disease. Then on January 21, 1993, he underwent resection of the tumor and associated enlarged lymph nodes. The pathology report indicates a largely necrotic, cystic tumor with an area of high-grade metastatic melanoma involving pelvic fibroadipose tissue and mesentery. A resected mesenteric nodule showed necrotic tissue and fibrosis largely replacing a mesenteric lymph node.

His surgeon, Dr. Turnbull, encouraged him to continue his nutritional program. After a lecture from me about the need for full compliance, Patient MW is again back on his full program, is again working full time and is in excellent health.

Patient MW is an informative case for a number of reasons. First, he has now completed more than five years on his nutritional protocol, with a history of recurrent melanoma that his Memorial physicians thought would kill him within months. Then, the documented changes in his tumor over the years illustrate a common occurrence for my patients with large masses. Initially, there was a period of slight growth, very common during the first six months or so of my therapy. I believe that this enlargement represents inflammation as the body seeks to control a tumor, rather than actual growth in malignant mass. Eventually the tumor stabilized before gradually turning into a cyst, an occurrence I associate with tumor death.

Unfortunately, after four years on his treatment, Patient MW felt so well he became overly confident, and completely disregarded the dietary part of his therapy, although he continued the supplements and the detoxification. The diet is as important as the other components, and not surprisingly his cancer began to grow quite rapidly. Clearly, although his tumor mass had been resolving over a four year period, he was not yet cured when he decided to ignore this dietary restrictions. In a sense, he represents his own control: on the full program, his disease slowly improved while off the protocol, his cancer worsened.

Dr. Gonzalez presented these 25 cancer case studies to the NCI in 1993 and then updated the patient status information in 2001. Below are Dr. Gonzalez's personal notes with updated survival information:

Metastatic stage IV melanoma. Alive and well 12 years out. This patient's survival status was updated again in 2016. Please refer to page 257 for this additional information.

THE MEDICAL CENTER OF DELAWARE
DEPARTMENT OF RADIOLOGY

Olin S. Allen II, M.D.	James Lally, M.D.	John T. Oglesby, M.D.	Leonard Rosenbaum, M.D.
S. Barry Diznoff, M.D.	S. Thomas Miller, M.D.	McHenry Peters, M.D.	Herman J. Stein, M.D.
Alan B. Evantash, M.D.	John L. McCormack, M.D.	Robert E. Price, M.D.	James H. Taylor, M.D.
John D. Kern, M.D.	Paul McCready, M.D.	Emanuel Renzi, M.D.	John S. Wills, M.D.
Zelimir Kozic, M.D.			

Patient Name :   M   W

Birth Date   :   11/18/31

Phone No.   :   444 1530

Date of Service : 5/16/88

X-Ray Number : 102696-8

Dear Dr. SAMII:

Following is the CAT SCAN OF THE ABDOMEN report on your
patient, W   M :

Computed axial tomographic images were obtained at 10mm
intervals through the abdomen and 20mm intervals through the
pelvis after the administration of oral contrast. No
intravenous contrast was given. Comparison is made with the
previous scans, the most recent dated 1/28/88. A 4.5 x 3.5cm
soft tissue mass has developed immediately anterior to the
spine slightly to the left of the mid-line at the level of the
aortic bifurcation. This is homogeneous soft tissue density
in appearance. There is some irregular soft tissue density
immediately superior to this to the left of the aorta which is
unchanged from previous scans and probably represents
residual fibrosis or unenlarged nodes. No enlarged abdominal
pelvis nodes are seen. No focal lesions are seen in the
liver, spleen, pancreas, kidneys, or gastrointestinal
structures. No bony lesions are seen. The findings are
consistent with local recurrence of patient's known melanoma.

IMPRESSION: RECURRENT 4.5 X 3.5CM SOFT TISSUE MASS IN THE
                   REGION OF AORTIC BIFURCATION CONSISTENT WITH
                   RECURRENT MELANOMA. NO ADENOPATHY OR OTHER
                   EVIDENCE OF METASTATIC DISEASE.

Thank you for referring this patient.

Sincerely,

THOMAS ZUNSTEG, M.D.
RESIDENT

JAMES F. LALLY, M.D.
RADIOLOGIST

JFL:cb
5/18/88 (1138

☐ c **Christiana Hospital** 4755 Ogletown-Stanton Road P.O. BOX 6001 NEWARK, DE 19718	☐ **Wilmington Hospital** 501 West 14th Street P.O. BOX 1668 WILMINGTON, DE 19899

3391 S (26540) (0887)   (302) 733 1800   (302) 428 2251

THE MEDICAL CENTER OF DELAWARE

DEPARTMENT OF RADIOLOGY

Olin S. Allen II, M.D.
S. Barry Diznoff, M.D.
Alan B. Evantash, M.D.
John D. Kern, M.D.
Zelimir Kozic, M.D.

James Lally, M.D.
S. Thomas Miller, M.D.
John L. McCormack, M.D.
Paul McCready, M.D.

John T. Oglesby, M.D.
McHenry Peters, M.D.
Robert E. Price, M.D.
Emanuel Renzi, M.D.

Leonard Rosenbaum, M.D.
Herman J. Stein, M.D.
James H. Taylor, M.D.
John S. Wills, M.D.

Patient Name : M. W.   Date of Service 9/7/88
Birth Date : 11/18/31   X-Ray Number 102696-8
Phone Number : 444-1530
Dear Dr. S. Samii:
cc:
Following is the CT SCAN OF THE ABDOMEN AND PELVIS report
on your patient, W. G. M.:

Computer tomographic images were obtained at 10 mm.
intervals through the abdomen and 20 mm. intervals through
the pelvis following oral and intravenous contrast
administration. The lung bases are clear. No pleural
effusion or pericardial abnormalities are present. No
metasatic lesions or other focal processes are seen within
the liver. No focal lesions are seen within the spleen,
adrenal glands or right and left kidneys. Left renal hilar
vascular calcifications are present. There is a large left
retroperitoneal mass near the aortic bifurcation as has
been previously described, and is again noted. On the last
CT scan performed on July 12, 1988, this mass measured
approximately 4 x 5 cm. in the AP and horizontal planes,
and on the current study it measures approximately 4.5 x 6
cm. respectively and, therefore, has slightly increased in
size. The previously described left periaortic adenopathy
and mesenteric adenopathy is not as evident on this
current study. The prostate gland is enlarged, but it is
homogeneous in attenuation. The pelvic structures are
otherwise normal.

IMPRESSION: 1. THERE IS NO EVIDENCE OF LIVER METASTASES.
                 THE   PREVIOUSLY   DESCRIBED   LEFT
                 RETROPERITONEAL SOFT TISSUE MASS HAS
                 SLIGHTLY INCREASED IN SIZE WHEN COMPARED
                 WITH THE PRIOR STUDY PREFORMED ON JULY
                 12, 1988.

Thank you for referring this patient.

                              SCOTT FARO, M.D.
                              RESIDENT

                              JAMES F. LALLY, M.D.
                              RADIOLOGIST

SF:ss(MB)
9/9/88

☑ Christiana Hospital
4755 Ogletown-Stanton Road
P.O. BOX 6001
NEWARK, DE 19718

☐ Wilmington Hospital
501 West 14th Street
P.O. BOX 1668
WILMINGTON, DE 19899

MEDICAL CENTER OF DELAWARE
DEPARTMENT OF RADIOLOGY

Olin S. Allen II, M.D.   James Lally, M.D.   John T. Oglesby, M.D.   Leonard Rosenbaum, M.D.
S. Barry Diznoff, M.D.   S. Thomas Miller, M.D.   McHenry Peters, M.D.   Herman J. Stein, M.D.
Alan B. Evantash, M.D.   John L. McCormack, M.D.   Robert E. Price, M.D.   James H. Taylor, M.D.
John D. Kern, M.D.   Paul McCready, M.D.   Emanuel Renzi, M.D.   John S. Wills, M.D.
Zelimir Kozic, M.D.

Patient Name : M   , W   Date of Service : 7-12-88
Birth Date   :   - 31   X-Ray Number   : 102696 8
Phone No.   :

_Dear Dr. S. Samii

Following is the CT ABDOMEN report on your patient, W
Me   :

Computed tomographic sections were obtained at 10 mm intervals
through the abdomen and 20 mm intervals through the pelvis.
Comparison is made to a previous recent scan dated 5-16-88. A
soft tissue mass near the aortic bifurcation present on that
study is again identified and the mass may be slightly larger
than previously, now measuring roughly 5 x 3.5 cm. There are
further changes since the previous studies; left para-aortic
adenopathy above the level of the bifurcation and below the
level of the left kidney is now thought to be present
(sections 19-22). Mesenteric adenopathy is also suggested to
the left of and anterior to the above described left
retroperitoneal nodes (sections 19-22). The large mass
described previously and now appearing slightly larger is in
continuity with the left retroperitoneal adenopathy
immediately above. There is slight fullness in the region of
the head of the pancreas but I believe this is produced by a
combination of vena cava, other vascular structures,
unopacified bowel, and head of the pancreas rather than being
due to pathology. No liver metastases are evident. No
adrenal metastases are identified. The lung bases appear
clear.

IMPRESSION: There has been a definite change since the study
of 5-16-88 with left retroperitoneal and probably left lower
mesenteric adenopathy now being present. Additionally, the
mass described previously in the low left retroperitoneum has
undergone slight further enlargement.

                              JOHN WILLS, M.D.
                              RADIOLOGIST

JSW:smc
July 13, 1988

☐   Christiana Hospital   ☐   Wilmington Hospital
     4755 Ogletown-Stanton Road   501 West 14th Street
     P.O. BOX 6001   P.O. BOX 1568
     NEWARK, DE 19718   WILMINGTON, DE 19899

18391 S (26540) (0588)   (302) 733-1800   (302) 428-2251

THE MEDICAL CENTER OF DELAWARE
DEPARTMENT OF RADIOLOGY

Olin S. Allen II, M.D.	James Lally, M.D.	John T. Oglesby, M.D.	Leonard Rosenbaum, M.D.
S. Barry Diznoff, M.D.	S. Thomas Miller, M.D.	McHenry Peters, M.D.	Herman J. Stein, M.D.
Alan B. Evantash, M.D.	John L. McCormack, M.D.	Robert E. Price, M.D.	James H. Taylor, M.D.
John D. Kern, M.D.	Paul McCready, M.D.	Emanuel Renzi, M.D.	John S. Wills, M.D.
Zelimir Kozic, M.D.			

Patient Name : M   , W.

Birth Date :   /31

Phone No. :

Date of Service : 12/22/88

X-Ray Number : 102696 8

cc: Nicholas J. Gonzalez, M.D.
737 Park Ave.
New York, N.Y. 10021

Dear Dr. Samii:

Following is the CT SCAN -- ABDOMEN AND PELVIS report on your
patient, W: .. M

Computed tomographic sections were obtained at 10 mm.
intervals through the abdomen and 20 mm. intervals through the
pelvis. 60 cc. of intravenous contrast were given at the
beginning of the study. Comparison is made to previous
studies, dated 9/7/68 and 7/11/88. A lower left retroperitoneal prominent mass, described on earlier scans, is
again identified and on section #24 where it appears largest,
it measures roughly 4.5 cm. in AP diameter by roughly 6 cm. in
width. This indicates little change in the size of this mass
since the previous study. Left retroperitoneal adenopathy
below the level of the renal hila, appreciated on the study
of 7/11/88, is not clearly seen at this time although there
remains some increase in soft tissue density in the area, not
well marginated, which could represent a residual of lymph
node enlargement or unopacified bowel loops here. No
mesenteric adenopathy is indicated on the current study. No
hepatic metastases are evident. No adrenal metastases are
suggested. There is an ovoid, roughly 1.5 cm. water density
lesion in the medial aspect of the lower pole of the right
kidney, seen also on some previous scans, felt likely to
represent an incidental renal cyst.

IMPRESSION: THE LOWER LEFT RETROPERITONEAL MASS DESCRIBED
PREVIOUSLY IS STILL EVIDENT AND HAS NOT CHANGED
SIGNIFICANTLY IN SIZE FROM THE STUDY OF 9/7/88.

Thank you for referring this patient.

Sincerely,

JOHN S WILLS, M.D.
RADIOLOGIST

JSW/sw
12/22/88 (1745)
c

☐ Christiana Hospital 4755 Ogletown-Stanton Road P.O. BOX 6001 NEWARK, DE 19718	☐ Wilmington Hospital 501 West 14th Street P.O. BOX 1668 WILMINGTON, DE 19899

18391 S (26540) (0887)   (302) 733-1800   (302) 428-2251   FILE

Olin S. Allen II, M.D.   James Lally, M.D.   John T. Oglesby, M.D.   Leonard Rosenbaum, M.D.
S. Barry Diznoff, M.D.   S. Thomas Miller, M.D.   McHenry Peters, M.D.   Herman J. Stein, M.D.
Alan B. Evantash, M.D.   John L. McCormack, M.D.   Robert E. Price, M.D.   James H. Taylor, M.D.
John D. Kern, M.D.   Paul McCready, M.D.   Emanuel Renzi, M.D.   John S. Wills, M.D.
Zelimir Kozic, M.D.

Patient Name   :   M.   , W.   Date of Service : 6/5/89
Birth Date   :   31   X-Ray Number   : 6/6/89
Phone No.   :   (3   1026968

Dear Dr. SIAMAK SAMII:

Following is the CAT SCAN OF THE ABDOMEN report on your
patient, W.   G. M   S:

Multiple enhanced computed tomographic scans were obtained in
the axial plane from the lung bases to the symphysis pubis.
Dilute barium was given by mouth to opacify bowel loops.
Comparison is made to previous CAT scan examinations, the most
recent being 12/22/88. The lung bases are clear. No
pulmonary parenchymal or pleural abnormality is identified.
The lower portion of the heart and pericardium appear normal
as well. The liver is normal in appearance without evidence
of focal abnormality. The spleen is unremarkable. Both
kidneys demonstrate normal symmetrical nephrograms. The
gallbladder is normal in appearance. No definite
abnormalities in the region of the pancreas are demonstrated.
There is poor contrast opacification of the proximal small
bowel. I see no dominant mass lesion within the proximal
mesentery but smaller lesions could easily be missed without
better bowel opacification. There has been no significant
change in the appearance of the mesenteric structures since
the previous examination. A dominant mass lesion is
demonstrated in the periaortic retroperitoneal soft tissues on
the left in the lower abdomen. This mass is best visualized
on scan sequence #24; it measures approximately 6cm transverse
by 4.2cm AP diamension. Its size and appearance has not
changed significantly since the previous examination. There
may be some residual lymphadenopathy in the periaortic
retroperitoneal soft tissues below the left renal hilum. Soft
tissue density in this area could also be caused by
unopacified bowel loops. However, the appearance in this
region has not changed significantly since the previous study
either. No definite mesenteric lymphadenopathy is visualized.
No definite iliac or inguinal lymphadenopathy is detected.
The protate gland appears slightly enlarged. The pelvic
structures are otherwise normal. The superficial soft tissues
of the abdominal and pelvic wall appear normal. Delayed scans
through the liver reveal no evidence of focal abnormality.

CONTINUED........

	Christiana Hospital		Wilmington Hospital
	4755 Ogletown-Stanton Road		501 West 14th Street
	P.O. BOX 6001		P.O. BOX 1668
	NEWARK, DE 19718		WILMINGTON, DE 19899

Olin S. Allen II, M.D.	James Lally, M.D.	John T. Oglesby, M.D.	Leonard Rosenbaum, M.D.
S. Barry Diznoff, M.D.	S. Thomas Miller, M.D.	McHenry Peters, M.D.	Herman J. Stein, M.D.
Alan B. Evantash, M.D.	John L. McCormack, M.D.	Robert E. Price, M.D.	James H. Taylor, M.D.
John D. Kern, M.D.	Paul McCready, M.D.	Emanuel Renzi, M.D.	John S. Wills, M.D.
Zelimir Kozic, M.D.			

Patient Name : M. ℞ W
Birth Date : 31
Phone No. :

Date of Service : 6/6/89
X-Ray Number : 6/6/89

PAGE TWO CONTINUED.......

IMPRESSION: MASS IN THE LEFT PERIAORTIC RETROPERITONEAL SOFT TISSUES IS UNCHANGED IN SIZE AND APPEARANCE SINCE 12/22/88. POSSIBILITY OF MINIMAL LEFT PERIAORTIC RETROPERITONEAL LYMPHADENOPATHY BELOW THE LEFT RENAL HILUM; THIS APPEARANCE HAS ALSO NOT CHANGED. NO OTHER ABNORMALITIES ARE DEMONSTRATED.

Thank you for referring this patient.

Sincerely,

RANDALL RYAN, M.D.
RADIOLOGIST

RR:cb
6/9/89 (0821)
DICT. 6/8/89
cc: NICHOLAS J. GONZALEZ, M.D.
737 PARK AVE.
NEW YORK, N.Y. 10021

☐ Christiana Hospital
4755 Ogletown-Stanton Road
P.O. BOX 6001
NEWARK, DE 19718

☐ Wilmington Hospital
501 West 14th Street
P.O. BOX 1668
WILMINGTON, DE 19899

18391 S (26540) (0588)   (302) 733-1800   (302) 428-2251   FILE

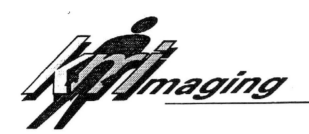

5509 kirkwood highway • wilmington, de 1980

Office 302/995-685
fax 302/995-967

November 14, 1990

Dr. J. Rooney
5500 Kirkwood Highway
Wilmington, DE 19808

Re: W   M.
MRI Pelvis
11/14/90

Age: 58
#MEA-3111

Dear Doctor Rooney:

MRI OF THE PELVIS

History: Low back and pelvic pain, previous abdominal tumor type unspecified.

Comment: MRI examination of the male pelvis was performed in a 0.06 Tesla Permanent Magnet. Coronal, sagittal and axial long TR/TE images were obtained. No short TR/TR images were obtained.

The study demonstrates that the images were obtained with a very large field of view making delineation of small abnormalities difficult. The lack of short TR/TE images also makes delineation of masses very difficult since it is difficult to characteristize any masses without short TR/TE images. For that reason, I would strongly suggest that this patient be brought back for repeat imaging of the pelvis as I suspect that there is a mass in the left rectosigmoid region. This mass may possibily be better studied with CT imaging since contrast can be administered. The mass is not clearly related to any solid organ. It is definitely not related to the prostate or bony structures of the pelvis. It is at the superior left aspect of the dome of the bladder. The mass appears to have a central portion which is of high signal intensity representing fluid or necrosis. Are any other studies available for review?

IMPRESSION: This study is suspicious for a LEFT SIDED PELVIC MASS which may be necrotic. Theoretically, this may be a loop of bowel filled with feces and fluid. A CT examination or comparison with previous studies is strongly suggested.

Incidnetally noted is severe degenerative disease involving the lumbar spine with bulging discs and possibile disc herniations of the lower lumbar spine. Further imaging is suggested if clinically indicated.

Very truly yours,

Philip Chao, M.D.

PC/de

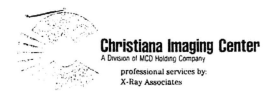

Christiana Imaging Center
A Division of MCD Holding Company

professional services by:
X-Ray Associates

X-ray and Ultrasound
Medical Arts Pavilion
at Christiana Hospital
Suite 107
4745 Ogletown-Stanton Road
Newark, Delaware 19713
(302) 731-9558

MRI CAT Scan Suite
4751 Ogletown-Stanton Roa
Newark, Delaware 19713
(302) 731-9800
Fax (302) 731-9088
Scheduling   MRI 731-986
CAT Scan 731-989

REFERRING PHYSICIAN: Siamak Samii, M.D.

PATIENT'S NAME: M. ʾɛ, W
FILM #:   C003002
DATE OF BIRTH: . . ʿ31

STUDY: CT of Abdomen/Pelvis
DATE OF SERVICE: 12/31/92

Dear Doctor:

Examination is performed at 10.0 mm. intervals through the abdomen and pelvis with comparison to a previous study from Christiana Hospital dated 6/6/89. Numerous Christiana Hospital studies are available to me; however, I have no CT study available performed more recently than June 1989.

The dominant abnormality is a roughly 7.0 cm. in diameter soft tissue mass in the left mid to lower pelvis, displacing the latter to the right and blending with nearby iliac vascular structures lateral to it on the left. This mass is heterogeneous showing both solid and apparently cystic or necrotic components. Dystrophic calcification is present as well. There was a mass present in this area on the previous scan and the mass has enlarged significantly since that time. There are several other abnormalities present; anterior to the lower inferior vena cava approximately 3.0 cm. above iliac crest level, there is a poorly marginated density measuring roughly 2.0 cm. in diameter and apparently containing curvilinear calcification peripherally. Although this could represent vascular structures and partially opacified bowel, the possibility of a small nodal mass with calcification is not excluded. In the left upper pelvis, a single loop of bowel is seen with a central small dot of contrast density, the overall appearance suggesting possible focal bowel wall thickening here. Mild right inguinal adenopathy is suggested. No other lymph node enlargement or mass is seen. No intestinal obstruction is evident. Incidental note is made of a probable small left renal artery aneurysm. Spleen size is normal and there are no focal hepatic or splenic lesions seen. No basilar lung abnormalities are evident.

Please see Page 2

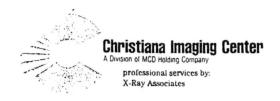

Christiana Imaging Center
A Division of MCD Holding Company

professional services by:
X-Ray Associates

X-ray and Ultrasound
Medical Arts Pavilion
at Christiana Hospital
Suite 107
4745 Ogletown - Stanton Road
Newark, Delaware 19713
(302) 731-9558

MRI CAT Scan Suite.
4751 Ogletown - Stanton Road
Newark, Delaware 19713
(302) 731-9800
Fax (302) 731-9088
Scheduling   MRI 731-9860
                CAT Scan 731-9890

Page 2

M̲⬚̲⬚̲ , W
C003002
CT-Abdomen/Pelvis
12/31/92

(Continued)

IMPRESSION: 7.0 CM. LEFT PELVIC MASS CONTAINING AREAS OF NECROSIS
AND CALCIFICATION AS DESCRIBED. THERE IS ALSO A
POSSIBLE SMALL MASS CONTAINING CALCIFICATION MEASURING
ROUGHLY 2.0 CM. IN DIAMETER IN THE RIGHT ABDOMEN
ANTERIOR TO THE INFERIOR VENA CAVA AT UMBILICAL LEVEL.
A SHORT SEGMENT OF POSSIBLE FOCAL SMALL BOWEL WALL
THICKENING IS NOTED AS WELL.

Thank you for referring this patient,

John S. Wills, M.D.
Radiologist

JSW/clc
January 11, 1993

ALAN D. TURNBULL, M. D.
1275 YORK AVENUE
NEW YORK. NEW YORK 10021
—
TELEPHONE 212 · 794-7562

September 21, 1987

Siamac Samii, M.D.
Medical Arts Pavilion
4745 Stanton Ogletown Road
Newark, Delaware 19713

Dear Doctor Samii: RE: W

This is to inform you that our mutual patient was discharged from Memorial
Sloan-Kettering Cancer Center September 20th following surgery 5 days earlier
for an obstructing mass involving his distal ileum and several adjacent loops
of small bowel. As you know, a percutaneously guided aspiration revealed
cells compatible with malignant melanoma and, at surgery, it was clear that
the patient's problem was due to massive adenopathy in the distal small bowel
mesentery invading several adjacent loops of bowel and rupturing to form a
contained cavity of necrotic tumor adjacent to the terminal ileum. The involved loops of bowel were resected with primary anastomosis but the pelvis
had seedings of tumor adjacent to the major mass   indicative of a drop
metastasis. For that reason and the fact that the tumor had ruptured and
subsequently become contained by the adjacent mesentery, it was felt appropriate only to "debulk" the mass, removing all but the capsule of tumor
against the sigmoid colon, base of mesentery, and posterior wall of the
bladder. There is minimal gross disease left in this patient's abdomen but,
since seedings had occurred and the tumor had ruptured prior to surgery, the
likelihood of diffuse melanomatosis is high.

Fortunately, Mr.   recovered bowel function without difficulty and had no
postoperative complications. At the beginning of the operative procedure Dr.
Elliot Strong performed a biopsy in the left nasal cavity and this was acute
inflammation with foreign body giant cell reaction only.

While in hospital the patient was seen by Dr. Dean Bajorin who is in charge
of our various melanoma research protocols including Interleukin-2, immunotherapy, etc. Dr. Bajorin reviewed what is available at our institution and
the results of standard and experimental therapy here and elsewhere. Mr. Mears
elected to take into consideration all that he had heard and to discuss these
options with his oncologists nearer to home. I look forward to seeing Mr.
         in follow up, perhaps alternating visits with Dr. Bajorin and Dr. Strong,
but at this moment am unclear as to what his follow up plans are. I think he
needs to digest what has been told to him, share it with his wife and discuss
these options with his internists at home. He has a very poor prognosis, a
tragedy in someone so young, courageous and knowledgeable. I only wish we
had more concrete options to present to him. His training as a scientist allows
him to understand our investigative protocols but also to realize that they are,
indeed, investigation only.

ALAN D. TURNBULL, M. D.
1275 YORK AVENUE
NEW YORK, NEW YORK 10021
—
TELEPHONE 212 - 794-7562

page 2
Siamac Samii, M.D.
September 21, 1987

It is my impression that Mr.   will be contacting me shortly regarding
his follow up plans and I will convey these to Dr. Strong. Should any additional information be needed, please do not hesitate to call me at the above
listed number.   A copy of the pathology report is enclosed.

Sincerely yours,

Alan D. Turnbull, M.D.
Associate Attending Surgeon
Memorial Sloan-Kettering Cancer Center

ADT/hlf
enc.
cc: Elliot Strong, M.D.
     Clifton Durning, M.D.
     J. McNally, M.D.

DESCRIPTION OF GROSS PATHOLOGY BY DR. ___Dr. Vuitch/lr_____ DATE ___11/30/84_____ 19 ___

#2. CLINICAL DIAGNOSIS: Malignant melanoma, left ethmoid sinus.
SOURCE OF TISSUE: Contents, left nasal cavity, septum, cribriform plate, lamina paparysia, orbit, and antral mucosa.

Received fresh are three pieces of tissue. The smaller two are bony with the larger of these, 1.0 cm, and are entirely submitted. The larger piece of tissue measures 7.5x6.8x4.0 cm in greatest dimension, and consists of a 6.0x4.0-cm portion of nasal septum, a 3.5x3.0-cm portion of cribriform plate, the left nasal cavity mucosa from the left cavity antrum, and a 2.5x3.3-cm portion of left lamina paparysia. On the left side of the superior portion of the nasal septum is a 5-mm focus of red soft tissue. Medial to the lamina popurysia is a 1.5-mm focus of blue and yellow firm tissue.

SUMMARY O F SECTIONS: A—Extra pieces of tissue—2; LNA—Left nasal antral mucosa—2; ANSM—Anterior nasal septal margin mucosa—2; INSM—Inferior nasal septal margin—2; AMM—Anterior maxilla margin—1; IMM—Inferior maxilla margin—1; PLRM—Posterior left nasal margin—1; PCM—Posterior cribriform margin—1; RCM—Right cribriform margin—1; ACM—Anterior cribriform margin—3; LLP—Left lamina pararysia—1; INT—Inferior nasal septal tissue—2; SNS—Superior nasal septal tissue—4; INSBM—Inferior nasal septal bony margin—2; ALNM—Anterior left nasal margin—1; ILNM—Inferior left nasal margin—1; LMM—Left maxillary margin—1; LSN—Left superior nasal tissue—1; LMS—Left mid nasal tissue—2; LIN—Left inferior nasal tissue—1; T—Possibel tumor—7; Total—43.

DR. S. BRUSTEIN/hva 12/3/84

3. CLINICAL DIAGNOSIS: MALIGNANT MELANOMA, LEFT ETHMOID SINUS
SOURCE OF TISSUE: LEFT SPHENOID MUCOSA

The specimen is received in formalin and consists of a fragment of edematous purple beige mucosa tissue measuring 2.5 x .7 x .3. Entirely submitted.

SUMMARY OF SECTIONS: Undesignated—1. Total 1.

4. CLINICAL DIAGNOSIS: MALIGNANT MELANOMA, LEFT ETHMOID SINUS
SOURCE OF TISSUE: FRAGMENT, LEFT POSTERIOR ETHMOID

The specimen is received in formalin and consists of an irregular mass of mucosal tissue and attached thin membraneous bone. The mucosal tissue measures 3 x 1 x .3 cm. The membraneous bone measures 1 x .7 x .1 cm. Entirely submitted.

SUMMARY OF SECTIONS: Undesignated—1. Decal—1. Total 2.

5. CLINICAL DIAGNOSIS: MALIGNANT MELANOMA, LEFT ETHMOID SINUS
SOURCE OF TISSUE: SPHENOID

The specimen is received in formalin and consists of an irregular thin membraneous tissue measuring 1.5 x 1 x .1 cm. Oriented into a small sac-like structure. Entirely submitted. SUMMARY OF SECTIONS: Undesignated—1. Total 1.

TION OF GROSS PATHOLOGY BY DR. _____ DR. S. BRUSTEIN/hva _____ DATE _____ 12/3/84 _____ 19

6.   CLINICAL DIAGNOSIS: MALIGNANT MELANOMA, LEFT ETHMOID SINUS
       SOURCE OF TISSUE: FRAGMENT LEFT ETHMOID MUCOSA

The specimen is feceived in formalin and consists of pink beige glistening
mucosal tissue, the larger fragment measures 2 x .7 x .2 cm. Entirely submitted.

SUMMARY OF SECTIONS: Undesignated— aggregate x 2.

7.   CLINICAL DIAGNOSIS: MALIGNANT MELANOMA, LEFT ETHMOID SINUS
       SOURCE OF TISSUE: POSTERIOR AND NASAL SEPTUM

The specimen is received in formalin and consists of two irregular fragments of
tissue, the largest fragment shows pink beige mucosa over cartilaginous tissue
and measures 2.5 x 2 x .7 cm. The second fragment is a small portion of mucosa.

SUMMARY OF SECTIONS: Undesignated—3.   Total 3.

9.   CLINICAL DIAGNOSIS: MALIGNANT MELANOMA, LEFT ETHMOID SINUS
       SOURCE OF TISSUE: RIGHT MIDDLE TURBINATE

The specimen is received in formalin and consists of an elongated portion of
mucosal tissue overlying cartilage and bone. The specimen measures 4 cm x .7 cm in
diameter.

SUMMARY OF SECTIONS: Decal—2.   Total 2.

10.   CLINICAL DIAGNOSIS: MALIGNANT MELANOMA, LEFT ETHMOID SINUS
        SOURCE OF TISSUE: RIGHT SPLENOID MUCOSA

The specimen is received in formalin and consists of an irregular purple beige
mucosal fragment measuring 1.5 cm in length by .7 x .2. Entirely submitted.

SUMMARY OF SECTIONS: Undesignated—1.   Total 1.

11.   CLINICAL DIAGNOSIS: MALIGNANT MELANOMA, LEFT ETHMOID SINUS
        SOURCE OF TISSUE: RIGHT SPLENOID SINUS

The specimen is received in formalin and consists of two irregular fragments of
purple beige glistening mucosal tissue, the larger fragment measures 2 x .7 x .2 cm.
Entirely submitted.

8.   CLINICAL DIAGNOSIS: MALIGNANT MELANOMA, LEFT ETHMOID SINUS
       SOURCE OF TISSUE: NASAL SPINE
The specimen is received in formalin and consists of five irregular small fragments
of bony tissue, the larger measuring .5 x .3 x .2 cm. Entirely submitted.

SUMMARY OF SECTIONS: DECAL—aggregate.   Total aggregate.

SURGICAL PATHOLOGY

SUBMITTED BY DOCTOR	_Turnbull_
SUBMITTED SLIDES ☐	SUBMITTED BLOCKS ☐
OUTSIDE SOURCE	

847067 M 55P

11595550 TURNBU

LABORATORY USE ONLY

☐ SMALL BIOPSY ☐ SPECIMEN ☐ SMEARS ☐ CLOT ☐ IMMEDIATE (EXAM (F.S.)

PATIENT NAME AND ADDRESS

1- FBI Lymph node ...

2- ...

3- p- Ileum Resected

10	11	12
8	9	

ANATOMIC SOURCE OF SPECIMEN _Abdomen_

CLINICAL DIAGNOSIS _Melanoma intra abdominal metastasis_

ACCESSION DATE AND NUMBER 14 SEP 87 18077

PREVIOUS ACCESSIONS IN THIS LABORATORY ☒ YES ☐ NO **PREVIOUS PATHOLOGY NUMBERS**

SIGNIFICANT CLINICAL DATA (USE ANATOMIC STAMPS WHEN POSSIBLE) AGE 55 SEX M

... 55 yr. ... resection 1974 ... Melanoma ... intra-abdominal mass ... liver ... recall ... elsewhere ...

DISPOSITION OF REPORT IF OTHER THAN CHART

PATHOLOGY REPORT

DATE OF REPORT 9/16/87 (SEE REVERSE SIDE FOR GROSS PATHOLOGY)

MICROSCOPIC REPORT BY DR. J. Woodruff/bpr

1- FROZEN SECTION: Benign
   PARAFFIN SECTION: Benign hyperplastic lymph node
2- FROZEN SECTION: Consistent with metastatic malignant melanoma.
   PARAFFIN SECTION: Metastatic malignant melanoma.
3- Metastatic melanoma involving mucosa, submucosa, and muscularis of a segment of small bowel. Melanoma also involves three mesenteric lymph nodes.
4- Acute inflammation with foreign body giant cell reaction.
5- Negative vermiform appendix.

1

(CONTINUED)

DESCRIPTION OF GROSS PATHOLOGY BY DR. __Dr. Heriot/ch_____ DATE __09/14/87____ 19 __

18077
#3.   CLINICAL DIAGNOSIS: Melanoma intra-abdominal metastasis
           SOURCE OF TISSUE: Resected ileum

Received fresh is a portion of small bowel which measures 14 x 12 x
7cm in greatest dimension. A single loop of small bowel measuring 32cm
long by up to 5.5cm wide is identified. The attached mesentery is
completely replaced by a tan firm tumor which measures 10 x 9 x 4cm.
When the bowel is opened, the circumference is 5.0cm. In the mid
portion of the specimen 9.0cm of the mucosa is replaced by a tan mass
which is continuous with the mesenteric mass. Thus, the mesenteric
mass appears to have eroded through the wall of the small bowel in the
central portion of the specimen. The remainder of the mucosa is
grossly unremarkable. The mucosa at the lines of resection is grossly
unremarkable.

SUMMARY OF SECTIONS: RM resection margins, 2; M mucosal tumor 2;
                     P. primary 2; LN lymph nodes 1
                                  Total 7
                     Dr.Prestipino/bpr   9/15/87

18077
5-   CLINICAL DIAGNOSIS: Melanoma, interabdominal metastasis
           SOURCE OF TISSUE: Appendix

The specimen is received in formalin and consists of a single
vermiform appendix that measures 8 cm. in length and has a maximum
diameter of approx. 1.5 cm. The appendix is serially sectioned
revealing the presence of an 8 cm. fecalith which irregularly dilates
the lumen of the appendix. There are no lesions noted on its serosal
surface or in the periappendiceal fatty soft tissues.

SUMMARY OF SECTIONS; Undes 3 total 3.

MEMORIAL SLOAN-KETTERING CANCER CENTER
1275 York Avenue, New York, NY 10021
212-639-5912, FAX# 212-717-3203

SURGICAL PATHOLOGY REPORT

Patient: **M** ,**W**	Accession #: **S93-1746**
MRN: 847067	Service:
Account #: 12662938	Date of Procedure: 01/21/93
DOB: Unknown (Age: 62) M	Date of Receipt: 01/21/93
Physician: Alan D. Turnbull, M.D.	Date of Report: 01/25/93

Clinical Diagnosis and History:
    METASTATIC MELANOMA

Specimens Submitted:
    Part 1: SP: MESENTERIC NODULE (FS) (M)
    Part 2: SP: PELVIC MASS (MC)
    Part 3: SP: RT ILIAC FOSSA LYMPH NODE (MC)

DIAGNOSIS:

1.   "MESENTERIC NODULE", EXCISION:
     - NECROTIC TISSUE SUGGESTIVE OF A METASTATIC NEOPLASM
     LARGELY REPLACING A FIBROTIC LYMPH NODE; CAN NOT IDENTIFY
     VIABLE TUMOR CELLS.

2.   "PELVIC MASS", EXCISION:
     - HIGH GRADE MALIGNANT NEOPLASM CONSISTENT WITH METASTATIC
     MALIGNANT MELANOMA INVOLVING FIBROADIPOSE TISSUE (THE TUMOR
     IS SIMILAR TO PREVIOUS-SEE 84-21648); TUMOR IS PRESENT AT
     SURGICAL MARGIN.

3.   LYMPH NODE, RIGHT ILIAC FOSSA, EXCISION:
     - ONE (1) LYMPH NODE, NO TUMOR SEEN.

Philip H. Lieberman, M.D./phl

** Report Electronically Signed Out **

Gross Description:
    (Giovanni Tallini, M.D./ggp)

1. Received in formalin, after frozen section, labeled "Mesenteric
Nodule," the specimen consists of a single nodule of yellow
necrotic tissue (1.5 x 1.5 x 1 cm.).

Summary of Sections:
FSC - Frozen Section Control
  U - Undesignated

** Continued on next page **   page 1

PATH.
REPORT
11

MEMORIAL SLOAN-KETTERING CANCER CENTER
1275 York Avenue, New York, NY 10021
212-639-5912, FAX# 212-717-3203

SURGICAL PATHOLOGY REPORT

Patient: M ,W
MRN: 847067

Accession #: **S93-1746**
Service:

Gross Description (continued):

2. Received fresh, labeled "Pelvic Mass, Metastatic Melanoma," the specimen consists of an 8 x 6 x 5.5 cm. mass of predominantly necrotic tumor tissue. The tumor is grossly present at the surgical margin, which is inked.

Summary of Sections:
U - Undesignated

3. Received in formalin, labeled "Lymph Node," is a single yellow portion of tissue (0.8 x 0.8 x 0.6 cm.) which is bisected and entirely submitted.

Summary of Sections:

Part	Sect. Site	Blocks	Pieces	All
1	FSC	1	1	Y
	U	3	3	
2	U	6	6	N
3	U	1	2	Y

Intraoperative Consultation:

Note: The diagnoses given in this section pertain only to the tissue sample examined at the time of the intraoperative consultation.

1. FROZEN SECTION DIAGNOSIS: NECROTIC TISSUE. (DF)
   PERMANENT DIAGNOSIS: SEE FINAL DIAGNOSIS.

** End of Report **

page 2

17. Patient NR
DOB: 3-16-34

Patient NR is a 59 year-old white Englishman with a history of recurrent melanoma. He had been in excellent health until July of 1990, when his wife noticed that a mole on his left ear had suddenly increased in size. Initially, Patient NR did not seek medical advice but when the lesion continued to grow, in January 1991 he went to his local physician who immediately referred him to a surgeon. On January 18, 1991, Patient NR underwent excision of the left ear lesion that proved to be melanoma, Clark's level IV, with 1.9 mm depth.

On January 28, 1991 Patient NR returned to surgery for a neck dissection, superficial parotidectomy and excision of the left ear in toto. Pathology studies revealed residual melanoma, depth to 1.2 mm. At the time, Patient NR was warned the disease might recur, but no additional treatment was recommended.

Patient NR did well until June of 1991, when he developed two nodules in the left mastoid area adjacent to the surgical incision site, as well as a nodule in the skin of the right axilla. A fine needle aspirate on June 26, 1991 confirmed metastatic melanoma; the three nodules were subsequently excised and all were found to be metastatic lesions. A full metastatic work-up in July 1991 included a normal chest X-ray as well as normal CT scans of the head, chest and abdomen. However, Patient NR's doctors advised him that his disease would eventually prove terminal, most likely within a year. As before, no further treatment with either chemotherapy or radiation was thought warranted.

Patient NR learned of my work and first came to my office on September 19, 1991. At that time, he felt well, was on no medications, and had a normal physical examination except for evidence of his extensive head and neck surgery.

Patient NR proved to be a very determined, and very compliant patient. When last seen on March 22, 1993, he was doing well, aside from fatigue from overwork and frequent air travel associated with his business activities. He has now completed nearly two years on his nutritional program, and remains in good health and apparently disease free.

Although I have no evidence of tumor regression for Patient NR while on my protocol, I thought him an interesting case to present. I have a series of patients with a history of recurrent melanoma that have done extremely well for periods of years without recurrence. For this aggressive disease, such long-term survival is unusual.

Dr. Gonzalez presented these 25 cancer case studies to the NCI in 1993 and then updated the patient status information in 2001. Below are Dr. Gonzalez's personal notes with updated survival information:

Metastatic melanoma. Alive and well 9 years out. This patient's survival status was updated again in 2016. Please refer to page 257 for this additional information.

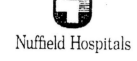

Nuffield Hospitals

FOR
Peter Millard

HISTOPATHOLOGY

LABORATORY No:- **910134**

DATE RECEIVED:-

	SPECIMEN:—
name N	
Name(s) R	*.... . .... LEFT*
D.B. 16.3.34 Sex M. Room No/OPD	*(Pinna)*
ddress WEAVERS Hs. INKPEN	
	PREVIOUS REPORT Nos.

FOR GYNAECOLOGICAL SPECIMENS	INVESTIGATION REQUIRED	
MP CYCLE	ROUTINE HISTOPATHOLOGY	☐
PARITY LAST PREGNANCY	RAPID HISTOPATHOLOGY	☑
HORMONAL TREATMENT YES / NO TYPE	FROZEN SECTION	☐

CLINICAL DETAILS AND DIAGNOSIS Small part ? melanoma
Left ear

DOCTOR PP M Godfrey DATE 18.1.91 ACCOUNT RENDERED TO DOCTOR / PATIENT

FOR LABORATORY USE ONLY

DESCRIPTION   BLOCKS

An ellipse of skin 1 x 0.5 x 0.2 cm bisected and all embedded.

HISTOLOGY: Within the central part the epidermis is partly ulcerated and within that
remaining there are increased numbers of infiltrating melanocytes. These cells are
often large with some pleomorphism amongst their nuclei and many include clear
cytoplasm. Within a few there is pigmentation within the cytoplasm. To either side of
this main lesion there are similar infiltrates and melanocytes within the epidermis.
Within the main lesion there is substantial cluster activity at the dermo-epidermal
junction of melanocytes and variably sized clusters of melanocytes lie within the
underlying dermis. At the base of this area a few melanocytes are more mature and
raise the possibility of an underlying benign naevus. There is also within this region
some increase in chronic inflammatory cells together with melanophages. None of the
changes extend to the lateral or to the deep margins of the section. The lesion is a
melanoma depth 1.9 mm and Clark's level 4.

SKIN: MELANOMA

P.R. Millard

<table>
<tr><td rowspan="2">DEPARTMENT OF HISTOPATHOLOGY
JOHN RADCLIFFE HOSPITAL
OXFORD
HISTOPATHOLOGY REPORT</td><td>Hospital No. ....
N:</td></tr>
<tr><td>Surname ....
R
First Names ....
16.03.34
Date of Birth .... Age................</td></tr>
</table>

PHYSICIAN or SURGEON   Mr Poole   WARD/DEPT.   Plastic Surgery

CLINICAL DATA   MM   left ear ? node left parotid.   Ear plus superficial parotid
    and left radical neck dissection.

SPECIMEN OF   Left ear and lesion from neck dissection (left)

SPECIMEN RECEIVED   29.01.91   REPORT DESPATCHED 4.2.91

REPORT

The entire left pinna 8 x 4 which includes a pigmented area, approximately
0.7 cm in the upper part.   Approximately 1.5 cm distal from this is a
small pigmented area.   This small pigmented area together with part of
the main lesion was given to Mr Stretch in the Plastic Surgery department.
Sections A and B - are residue of the pigmented lesion.   Attached is a
fibromuscular mass 16 x 11 x 3 cm.   The was finely diced and any lymph
nodes sectioned and embedded.   Section C - includes salivary glands.

HISTOLOGY

Within the region of the pigmented lesion there are groups of melanocytes
lying mainly within the dermis, sometimes approaching the dermoepidermal junction
and occasionally in clumps at the dermoepidermal junction as well as infiltrating
into the epidermis.   The latter changes often more apparent within hair follicles.
The melanocytes exhibit pleomorphism and dysplasia and are mainly cuboidal
in type. Most have clear cytoplasm but within a few there is pigment compatible
with melanin within the cytoplasm.   The cells are arranged in small groups
and islands as well as in intervening strands and lying individually.   There
is some fibrosis within parts of the tumour, probably in response to the previous
surgery, together with some lymphocytic and neutrophil polymorph infiltrate.
The infiltrated tumour is markedly vascular and the possibility of vascular
invasion cannot be ruled out.   The tumour does not extend to the underlying
cartilage in any of the sections.   The maximum tumour depth is 1.2 mm.   No
tumour is evident within the 3 lymph nodes identified within the attached
tissue and no tumour is evident within the salivary gland also included with
this tissue.

EAR - MELANOMA.
LYMPH NODES - REACTIVE CHANGES.

Signature. ....

Dr P R Millard

LABORATORY NO. | NATURE OF SPECIMEN
Pl melanoma (Ler
 $m \sim$ nodule regio
 mastoid $\sim Ym$.

Collection date 2?/6/91 .... and time 16)()

INVESTIGATION REQUIRED   cytology

MHS	BTA	JP
Primary		OF
Coll	Other	TC

CLINICAL DETAILS:
(Mention Chemotherapy, with Dates
and Date of Onset of Disease)

SIGNATURE

When filling in Request Cards
PLEASE
1. Give ALL the relevant information requested.
2. Use BLACK ink (for clear photocopying)
3. Complete a separate card for EACH specimen.

PATHOLOGY REQUEST	Date Received
	2?/6/91

AB4.44.9 3

FC DATE   : 26.6.91   LAB NUMBER : NG 91/1087P

NAME   : N   R

SPECIMEN   : FNA Lymph Node

DIAGNOSIS   : Many malignant cells present, morpho-
                  logically consistent with metastatic
                  malignant melanoma.

SIGNED   : WG

DATE OF REPORT : 28.6.91

DEPARTMENT OF HISTOPATHOLOGY	Hospital No. 1208299
JOHN RADCLIFFE HOSPITAL	Surname N.
OXFORD	First Names R .
HISTOPATHOLOGY REPORT	Date of Birth 16.3.1934 Age

PHYSICIAN or SURGEON Mr Poole   WARD/DEPT. Plastics.

CLINICAL DATA   Melanoma left ear 1991.   Now nodule under nearby skin and
in right arm.

SPECIMEN OF   Lesion 1. upper mastoid, 2. lower mastoid, 3. lesion in
upper right arm.

SPECIMEN RECEIVED   1.7.91   REPORT DESPATCHED   4.7.91

REPORT

1. Portion of skin measuring 1.6 x 1 cm with underlying deep tissue 0.4 cm.
The surface shows three small pigmented areas. Serially sliced, all embedded
in one cap.

2. There are two fragments of fatty connective tissue, the largest measuring
2 x 1.5 x 0.3 cm and the smaller 1.1 x 1 x 0.2 cm. There is no obvious skin
surface. The larger fragment is serially sliced and all embedded in two caps,
A/B, the smaller fragment all embedded in cap C.

3. Skin ellipse 2 x 1 cm with underlying fatty tissue 1.5 x 2 x 1.5 cm. There
are obvious dark pigmented areas within the fatty tissue. Serially sliced,
all embedded in four caps.

HISTOLOGY

1. Sections show fibro fatty connective tissue embedded in which are two lymph
nodes. The normal lymph node architecture has been totally effaced and replaced
by metastatic tumour. The tumour cells show nuclear pleomorphism with prominent
nucleoli and have fairly abundant eosinophilic cytoplasm. There is
of the tumour cells and the histological appearances would be compatible with
metastatic melanoma.

2. Sections show fibro fatty connective tissue embedded in which is a single
lymph node. This too has been largely replaced by the same metastatic tumour.

3. Sections show a portion of skin together with underlying dermis and subcutaneous
fat. Within the subcutaneous fat are at least 6 lymph nodes, all of which
have been largely replaced by metastatic tumour consistent with primary melanoma.

1, 2 & 3. LYMPH NODES IN REGION OF UPPER MASTOID, LOWER MASTOID AND INNER
UPPER RIGHT ARM: METASTATIC MELANOMA.

Signature
Dr C Baierie/Dr P R Millard

Ovarian Cancer

18. Patient SD
DOB: 12/9/49

Patient SD is a 43 year-old white woman with a long history of ovarian cancer. In early 1982, she first developed abdominal bloating and discomfort. After a gynecological work-up, on March 29, 1982 at Beth Israel Hospital in New York she went for exploratory surgery, right oophorectomy and partial left oophorectomy. The pathology report documents papillary serous cystadenocarcinoma, felt to be of low malignant potential. At the time no additional therapy was recommended. Initially, Patient SD did well, but within six months she developed ascites and underwent paracentesis. The fluid cytology was positive, and in August, 1983 she underwent total abdominal hysterectomy and left salpingo-oophorectomy for extensive pelvic disease. She was subsequently followed with repeat laparoscopies, and in 1984, Patient SD received a course of P-32 because of persistent cancer cells in ascitic fluid.

For several years, she seemed to stabilize but then on August 8, 1988 a pelvic ultrasound revealed a right lower quadrant abdominal wall mass. Needle biopsy confirmed metastatic cancer, and on September 9, 1988, Patient SD returned to surgery for resection of the mass along with multiple pelvic nodules. All visible tumor was excised. However, less than six months later, in February 1989, Patient SD developed an enlarged left supraclavicular lymph node. On February 24, 1989, the node was aspirated—not resected—and cytology studies proved positive for recurrent malignancy. At this point chemotherapy was suggested but refused by the patient.

Patient SD learned of my work and first came to see me on May 17, 1989. At that time, she felt well. She was on no medications. Her examination was notable for several 1 cm, hard, non-tender left cervical nodes.

Shortly after her initial visit, Patient SD began her nutritional protocol which she followed enthusiastically. After she completed two years on her therapy, a CT scan of the abdomen and pelvis performed February 4, 1991 showed no evidence of disease. Her cervical nodes have remained stable on examination and when last seen on May 7, 1993, she was in excellent health, and planning to get married. She has now completed more than four years on her nutritional regimen, with apparent control of her once progressing malignancy.

Dr. Gonzalez presented these 25 cancer case studies to the NCI in 1993 and then updated the patient status information in 2001. Below are Dr. Gonzalez's personal notes with updated survival information:

Stage IV ovarian cancer. Quit the program after 4 years. I understand she is alive.

DEPARTMENT OF PATHOLOGY
AMERICAN ONCOLOGIC HOSPITAL -- JEANES HOSPITAL
PHILADELPHIA, PENNSYLVANIA 19111
Report of Tissue or Cell Morphology

Patient: S   , D   Case No:
Room No: OPD   Age: 49 36 years   Spec No: SO-86-3678
Physician: Hogan   Date: 08/22/1986

Pre-op Diag:
Post-op Diag:
History:
Specimen: Slide Review: Beth Israel Medical Center,
              10 Nathan D. Perlman Place, N.Y., N.Y. 10003,
              Slide No. S82-4231 (9), S82-14713 (2), S83-7182 (2), S83-10633
              (26).

GROSS DESCRIPTION: Received are a total of 39 microscopic slides. They are
received from Beth Israel Medical Center.

MICROSCOPIC DESCRIPTION: Some of the slides are labelled 82S-4231 and the
accompanying report identifying the exact source of the tissue on these
slides is not present. There is a supplementary report provided which implies
that at least some of the slides show a right ovarian neoplasm as well as a
peritoneal implant. Review of some of these slides reveal a papillary
epithelial neoplasm of the ovary. There are stalks composed of vascular
fibrous connective tissue that are covered with epithelium, which is heaped up
in several cell layers in some areas. Mitoses are rare, and atypia of the
epithelial cells is not great. No actual invasion of the underlying stroma is
seen. One section shows similar appearing papillary structures invading
fibrous connective tissue. Psammoma bodies are a prominent feature in this
tissue, and this finding of invasiveness is most consistent with low grade
malignant potential. Therefore, it is felt that the papillary neoplasm
represented in these slides is a papillary serous cystadenocarcinoma of low
malignant potential. Two slides are labelled S-82-14713. According to the
accompanying report, these represent biopsies of the right round ligament and
tissue from the cul-de-sac. Review of these slides reveal metastatic implants
of papillary serous cystadenocarcinoma. Two of the slides are labelled S-83-
7182. According to the accompanying report, this represents tissue taken from
the left and right ovaries. The section showing tissue from the left ovary
reveals a papillary, serous, cystadenoma having features consistent with
borderline malignancy. Review of the second slide reveals fragments of
epithelial tumor similar in appearance, including psammoma bodies. Most of
these fragments are within fibrous connective tissue. No definite ovarian
tissue is identified. The remaining 26 slides are labelled 83S-10633. The
slide sublabelled 1, representing endocervical curettings, contains no tissue.
A slide sublabelled 2, representing endometrial curettings, shows benign
proliferative endometrium. A slide sublabelled 3, representing an old scar,
reveals dermal fibrosis consistent with cicatrix. The slide sublabelled 4,
represent the right adnexa. These show fallopian tube containing a
metastatic, papillary, serous, epithelial neoplasm containing many psammoma
bodies. Sections of the uterus and cervix show adenomyosis, benign
proliferative endometrium and chronic cystic cervicitis. Sections of the left
fallopian tube and left ovary show a papillary, serous cystadenoma of
borderline malignancy with psammoma bodies. A similar tumor is found in the
left fallopian tube. Implants are found on the serosal surface of the uterus.
Implants are also seen in sections from the cul-de-sac and omentum. No slides
from the tissue labelled adhesions of bowel are available for review.

Page 1
(Continued on following page)

DEPARTMENT OF PATHOLOGY
AMERICAN ONCOLOGIC HOSPITAL -- JEANES HOSPITAL
PHILADELPHIA, PENNSYLVANIA 19111
Report of Tissue or Cell Morphology

Patient: S   D   Case No:
Room No: OPD   Age: 12/9/1949 36 years   Spec No: SO-86-3678
Physician: Hogan   Date: 08/22/1986

DIAGNOSIS: Ovarian mass (S82-4231) - papillary, serous, cystadenocarcinoma of
             low malignant potential, with invasive peritoneal implant.

             Biopsy of right round ligament (S82-14713) - metastatic implants
             of papillary cystadenocarcinoma of low malignant potential.

             Tissue from cul-de-sac (S82-14713) - metastatic implant of
             papillary cystadenocarcinoma of low malignant potential.

             Left ovarian tissue (S83-7182) - papillary, serous, cystadenoma of
             borderline malignancy.

             Right ovarian tissue (S83-7182) - fragments of papillary, serous,
             cystadenoma of borderline malignancy within fibrous
             connective tissue.

             Left adnexal mass (S83-10633) - papillary, serous, cystadenoma of
             borderline malignancy within fibrous connective tissue.

             Left adnexal mass (S83-10633) - papillary, serous, cystadenoma of
             borderline malignancy.

             Right and left fallopian tubes (S83-10633) - serosal surfaces with
             multiple tumor implants and psammoma bodies, mucosa of
             fallopian tubes containing psammoma bodies.

             Uterus (S83-10633) - proliferative endometrium, adenomyosis,
             chronic cystic cervicitis, serosal surface with implants.

             Cul-de-sac (S83-10633) - serosal implants containing psammoma
             bodies.

             Segment of omentum (S83-10633) - omentum containing multiple
             papillary epithelial tumor implants with psammoma bodies.

Michael J. Kowalyshyn, M.D.

MJK:rgh   (4-SEP-86 14:05:16)

This case has been reviewed by and with:
Codes: 87000 84603   18010 84603   44590 84603   87020 84603
          87010 84603   86120 84603   86120 84603   86800 55590
          82000 76000   82000 76510   82000 40000   Y4590 55590
          63850 55590

BETH ISRAEL MEDICAL CENTER

FIRST AVENUE AT 16TH STREET, NEW YORK, NY 10003

PATIENT	MEDICAL RECORD NO	DATE OF SURGERY
SEAF~ D		9/27/88

SURGEON	ASSISTANTS
DR. WALLACH, DR. CONRAD	DR. SHU, DR. NABATIAN.

PREOPERATIVE DIAGNOSIS: RECURRENT BORDERLINE OVARIAN TUMOR.

POSTOPERATIVE DIAGNOSIS: SAME (PATHOLOGY PENDING).

ANESTHESIA: GENERAL ENDOTRACHEAL INTUBATION.

OPERATION: 1. VAGINAL VAULT IMPLANTS BIOPSY, FOR FROZEN SECTION. 2. DIAGNOSTIC LAPAROSCOPY. 3. EXPLORATORY LAPAROTOMY. 4. ABDOMINAL WALL MASS *Excision* INCISION. 5. MULTIPLE PELVIC NODULES EXCISION BIOPSY. 6. PARTIAL OMENTECTOMY.

FINDINGS:
There are two tiny vaginal vault implants and frozen section shows vaginal mucosa only. The diagnostic laparoscopy revealed that there is 100 cc fluid in the cul-de-sac area (yellowish-green) and there is a 4x3x3 abdominal wall mass over the right lower quadrant area. One nodule was noted on sigmoid and another one was on right pelvic sidewall. There are three nodules over cul-de-sac and with outer wall area. Exploratory laparotomy – the findings of the abdominal wall mass was between muscle and peritoneal layer. The mass measures 4 cm. The right pelvic wall mass and the epiploic of sigmoid colon, cul-de-sac and bladder and bladder wall nodules wall and radical excision biopsy of the nodules.

Estimated blood loss: 600 cc.
Specimen: 1. vaginal vault biopsy. 2. Peritoneal fluid cytology. 3. Abdominal wall mass. 4. abdominal mass. 5. Mass of the sigmoid. 6. Right IP ligament mass. 7. Right pelvic sidewall mass. 8. Right round ligament mass. 9. A.P.E.P. 10. Bladder tail. 11. Left cul-de-sac mass. 12. omentum #1. 13. Omentum #2. 14. Omentum #3.

Closure: 0 chromic for the peritoneal,. 0 PDS for the fascial layer and 00 plain for the subcutaneous, 4-0 Vicryl for the skin.
Complications: None.

PROCEDURE:
The patient was brought to the Operating Room and placed int the supine position. After the induction of general intubation with endomtracheal tube, the patient was repositioned to the frogleg position. Vaginal speculum was then inserted into the vagina. There two small implants were noted on the five and seven o'clock area of the vaginal vault. Excision biopsys were

BETH ISRAEL MEDICAL CENTER

FIRST AVENUE AT 16TH STREET, NEW YORK, NY 10003

	MEDICA'	DATE OF SURGERY
: D : T		
	ASSISTANTS	

page 2

performed with scalpels. The specimen was sent to Pathology
for frozen section. The frozen section report showed vaginal
mucosa only. Then Monsel Solution was applied to the incisional
area for hemostasis. Then the Foley catheter was inserted under
sterile conditions. The patient was repositioned to the supine
position and the patient was then prepped and draped in sterile
condition for laparoscopy.

Next, a 1 cm periumbilical incision was made with the first scalpel.
A hemostat was used for the blunt dissection down to the fascial
layer. The Lahey retractors were used to elevate the skin to
expose the fascia. The fascia was then entered bluntly with
the hemostat and extended bluntly with the hemostat. The Lahey
retractors were then repositioned to elevate the fascia to the
skin to expose the parietal peritoneum. The parietal peritoneum
was then grasped with two hemostats and tented and nicked wit
the scalpel. The peritoneum was then extended bluntly with the
hemostat.

Lahey retractors then repositioned to elevate the peritoneum,
fascia and skin. Next, the blunt trocar with sleeve was inserted
through the skin incision into the peritoneal cavity. The blunt
trocar was then removed and laparoscope inserted and revealed
that we were within the peritoneal cavity. Carbon dioxide gas
was then insufflated into the peritoneal cavity to create a
pneumoperitoneum.

Next, under direct laparoscopy visualization, a Verres needle
was then pushed into the peritoneal cavity and over the suprapubic
site. On examination of pelvic organs, the uterus and the bilateral
adnexa were absent due to previous hysterectomy and salpingo-
oophorectomy for borderline ovarian tumor. There is a 100 cc
of yellowish-green fluid in the cul-de-sac area and 4x3x3 cm
abdominal wall mass over right lower quadrant area. One nodule
was noticed on the sigmoid colon and the one was found on the
right pelvic sidewall.

There is a whitish-gray area of nodules which are located between
the infundibulopelvic ligament and the round ligament stump.
There are three nodules, one is over the cul-de-sac area and
bladder wall. The liver, spleen and diaphragm are exposed.
NO nodules noted. Then the cul-de-sac area fluids were suctioned
out with syringe connected to the Verres needle. About 80 cc
of yellowish fluid was collected. Specimen was sent for cytology.

Then the laparoscope was removed from the sleeve and the blunt
trocar was inserted back into the sleeve and together the sleeve

BETH ISRAEL MEDICAL CENTER

FIRST AVENUE AT 16TH STREET, NEW YORK, NY 10003

	MEDICAL RECORD NO.	DATE OF SURGERY
...AFF... , D...		
...ON	ASSISTANTS	

page 3

and the blunt trocar were withdrawn from the peritoneal cavity.
Then the fascial layer and the periumbilical incision was closed
with figure-of-eight suture of 0 chromic. Skin was closed with
000 plain catgut.

Then we started to perform the exploratory laparotomy. A 5 cm
small righrt low transverse skin incision was made with scalpels.
Subcutaneous bleeders were clamped and tied with 00 plain. The
fascia was nicked and the fascial incision was extended laterally
to the right and midline using the Metzenbaum scissors. THen
abdominal wall mass which measured 4x3x3 cm, firm, nodular were
palpable between the rectus muscle and peritoneal layers and
one nodule which measured 0.5x0.5 cm was palpable over the lateral
pelvic walls and irregular surface palpable over right pelvic
walls which was located between infundibulopelvic ligament and
the round ligament stump area.

At this time, Dr. Wallach attended to the Operating Room and
suggested to remove the abdominal wall mass with partial rectus
muscle removal. The right rectus muscle was separated layer
by layerwith clamps and then dissected and tied with 0 chromic.
Then the abdominal wall mass with partial rectus muscle was removed
and then bleeders were secured. At this time, one yellowish
green nodule which measured 0.5 cm was found over the sigmoid
colon.

An Allis clamp was used to grasp the nodule and clamp was placed
between the nodule and the sigmoid colon. The nodule was removed
with staples. Then another 0.5 cm nodule was found over the
right vaginal pelvic sidewall. The nodule was removed with the
same procedure. Then because the right pelvic sidewall nodule
between the infundibulopelvic ligament and the round ligament
was palpable and there are multiple nodules over the bladder
wall and epiploic of the colon and the cul-de-sac area, we decided
to extend the skin incision.

The incision was extended with a knife. The bleeders were clamped
and tied with 00 plain. Then the fascia was extended laterally
to the left using the Metzenbaum scissors. The bowels were packed
away with two moist lap pads. A right angle retractor was placed
to give good visual field because the whitish irregular nodules
which are located between the IP ligament and the round ligament
were close to right ureter and Dr. Wallach decided to open peritoneum.
The retroperitoneum was picked up and incised with Metzenbaum
scissors and then right ureter was visualized and peristalsis

BETH ISRAEL MEDICAL CENTER

FIRST AVENUE AT 16TH STREET, NEW YORK, NY 10003

PATIENT	MEDICAL RECORD	DATE OF SURGERY
D		
SURGEON	ASSISTANTS	

page 4

was noted. Then a vessel was found above the ureter. The vessel
was clamped, dissected and tied. Then the whitish nodule was
removed. Grossly is suspect for tumor mass of the IP ligament
stump granulation tissue. Then the ureter was carefully separated
above tunnel with Adson clamp. Then the ureter was clearly identified.
The whitish nodule around the round ligament stump was carefully
removed.

Then the fascia reperitonealized with 00 chromic performed.
Then attention was paid to the cul-de-sac and bladder wall area.
The left sigmoid colon adhedsins to the bladder wall. Careful
lysis of adhesions was then performed with Metzenbaum scissors.
There two yellowish-green nodules were noted. These nodules
were removed with Metenbaum scissors nad the stumps were tied
with 0 chromic. The nodules were also noted on the cul-de-sac
area and the bladder wall.

These nodules were removed in the same way. Then hemostasis
was secured. Then the partial omentectomy was performed with
two clamps and dissected and tied with 0 chromic tie. then the
pelvic cavity was completely examined by Dr. Wallach and Dr.
Conrad. No residual tumor was left. We then decided to close
the abdomen in the following way.

The peritoneum was closed using running 0 chromic suture. The
fascia was closed using an interlocking figure-of-eight 0 PDS.
The subcutnaeous tissue was reapproximated with 000 plain and
the skin was closed with 4-0 Vicryl and Steri-Strips. The patient
was then awakened from the general endotracheal anesthesia and
taken to the Recovery Room in stable condition.

DICTATED BY DR. SHU
S/lvs/RR
c: 332
T: 9/29/88 D: 9/28/88

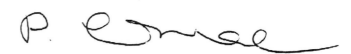

THE LANKENAU HOSPITAL   PHILA., PA.
IRWIN K. KLINE, MD., CHM., DEPT OF PATHOLOGY

CYTOLOGY REPORT

NAME: S   ,D   ACC. NO.:

MED. REC. NO.: 653520
BIRTHDATE: 12/09/1949   AGE/SEX: 39Y F

LOCATION: OP   PHYSICIAN: HOGAN, W. MICHAEL

DATE COLLECTED: 02/24/89
DATE RECEIVED: 02/27/89

SPECIMEN: LT CERV NODE, N.A.

RESULTS: POSITIVE
        CELLS COMPATIBLE WITH METASTATIC CARCINOMA WITH
        GLANDULAR AND FOCAL PAPILLARY FEATURES. THIS MAY
        BE FROM PREVIOUS OVARIAN CARCINOMA, HOWEVER A
        PRIMARY BREAST CARCINOMA SHOULD ALSO BE
        CONSIDERED.

                REVIEWED BY: T. S. KLINE, M.D.
                             VAIDEHI KANNAN, M.D.

PATIENT FIRST NAME: L ___   LAST NAME: S.
RECORD NUMBER   : MR077942   BIRTH DATE: /1949
RADIOLOGIST: Michael Clair   REFERRING PHYSICIAN(s): Dr Hogan

STUDY NAME: CT OF ABDOMEN AND PELVIS   STUDY DATE: 02/04/1991
HISTORY: Ovarian CA.

COMMENT: Comparison is made with the prior study of 2 June, 1989. There
is no definite measurable disease. There are small retroperitoneal
and pelvic lymph nodes, none of which demonstrates any interval increase
in size. A 1 cm. left subdiaphragmatic nodule is present on image #13
which was not definitely present but is of doubtful significance without
evidence of other measurable disease. Lymph nodes in the root of the
mesentery are prominent but unchanged. There is no evidence of hdro-
nephrosis. CT scanning of the pelvis demonstrates no abnormalities.
There may be a tiny 5 to 10 mm. left adnexal/ovarian cyst. This is of
doubtful significance.

IMPRESSION: No definite measurable tumor and no essential change
from June 1989.

Pancreatic Cancer

19. Patient: SM
DOB: 6/9/21

Patient SM is a 72 year-old white male with a history of metastatic adenocarcinoma of the lung. He has a history of heavy cigarette smoking, but otherwise had been in good health when in July of 1991, a right pulmonary nodule was noted on a routine chest X-ray. Patient SM's physician referred him for a complete metastatic work-up: a CT scan of the chest on August 20, 1991 confirmed a 6 mm. nodule in the right upper lobe, associated with a mildly enlarged mediastinal node. A CT of the brain on September 6, 1991 was negative, but a CT of the abdomen the same date revealed four lesions of the right lobe of the liver, a round enlargement of the right adrenal gland up to 2 cm. in size, diffuse enlargement of the left adrenal, and a 4.5 cm. mass in the porta hepatis or upper pancreatic head. Ultrasound on September 24, 1991 documented areas consistent with metastatic disease in the liver, the largest measuring 3.4 to 4 cm. near the hilus, the second just under 2 cm. in the right lobe, and possibly a third smaller lesion in the right lobe. Bone scan showed increased uptake in the right shoulder and right hip.

On September 24, 1991, he underwent mediastinoscopy, right thoracotomy and excision of the right upper lobe nodule. Mediastinal nodes were negative for disease, but the right upper lobe nodule was found to be infiltrative moderately differentiated adenocarcinoma. Because of the extensive disease at the time of diagnosis, patient SM was told he had terminal disease, and neither chemotherapy nor radiation were recommended. In September of 1991, while being evaluated, he began an intensive nutritional protocol under his own direction. I first saw patient SM on December 12, 1991 and at the time he had no complaints, despite the aggressive nature of his disease. He was on Calan SR, Hydralazine, Amiloride/HCT and KDur for hypertension, as well as multiple nutritional supplements. His exam was notable for psoriatic lesions. Blood work was unremarkable, including normal liver function tests.

Patient SM began my therapy in December of 1991 with great determination. Today, he remains generally very compliant except for occasional dietary indiscretions, and is nearly two years out from his original diagnosis. He is in excellent health with no complaints and leads a very active life in a Florida retirement community.

Interestingly, a CT scan of the abdomen on February 4, 1993—when patient SM was 18 months out from diagnosis—revealed virtually no change in any of the lesions. This is not an unusual occurrence with my protocol: frequently, tumors gradually regress and resolve but almost as commonly, repeat radiographic studies over a period of years show no change in tumors. I suspect in these latter patients, the body gradually walls off areas of cancer, replacing malignant lesions with fibrotic tissue and inflammatory debris. Such patients do as well clinically as those in whom we document obvious tumor regression.

Dr. Gonzalez presented these 25 cancer case studies to the NCI in 1993 and then updated the patient status information in 2001. Below are Dr. Gonzalez's personal notes with updated survival information:

Metastatic pancreatic cancer. Alive and well 9 years out. No sign of disease.

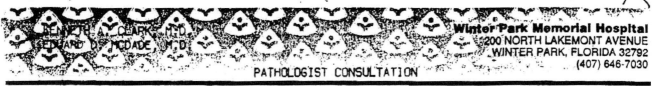

Winter Park Memorial Hospital
200 NORTH LAKEMONT AVENUE
WINTER PARK, FLORIDA 32792
(407) 646-7030

PATHOLOGIST CONSULTATION

NAME: S.   M.   ROOM: ICU /ICU - 5   PATH #:

HOSP#:   AGE: 70 YRS   DOB: 21   SEX: M   RACE: WHITE

DATE TAKEN: 09/24/91   DATE RECV'D: 09/25/91   DATE REPT: 09/25/91

PHYSICIAN: ROBINSON, HUGH B.   SURGEON: ROBINSON, HUGH

MATERIAL SUBMITTED: 1. SUBCARINAL LYMPH NODE FOR FROZEN SECTION
                     2. RIGHT PARATRACHEAL LYMPH NODE FOR FROZEN SECTION
                     3. MEDIASTINAL LYMPH NODES X 3 FOR FROZEN SECTION
                     4. RIGHT UPPER LOBE NODULE FOR FROZEN SECTION

CLINICAL HISTORY: MULTIPLE LESIONS SUGGESTIVE OF METASTATIC DISEASE

DIAGNOSIS:
----

1. SUBCARINAL LYMPH NODES, BIOPSY: NEGATIVE FOR NEOPLASM.

2. RIGHT PARATRACHEAL LYMPH NODE, BIOPSY: NEGATIVE FOR NEOPLASM.

3. MEDIASTINAL LYMPH NODE, BIOPSY: NEGATIVE FOR NEOPLASM.

4. RIGHT UPPER LOBE LUNG NODULE, BIOPSY: INFILTRATIVE MODERATELY
                              DIFFERENTIATED ADENOCARCINOMA.
TC2

                    Kenneth A. Clark, M.D.
                    ------------------------------ 09/25/91
                    Pathologist   (electronic signature)

MACROSCOPIC DESCRIPTION:
----

1. LABELLED "SUBCARINAL LYMPH NODE". THERE ARE THREE PIECES OF BLACK AND
RED TISSUE INDIVIDUALLY MEASURING UP TO 0.5 CM IN GREATEST DIMENSION. ALL
EMBEDDED.

FROZEN SECTION DIAGNOSIS: NEGATIVE FOR NEOPLASM.   KAC/LMF

2. LABELLED "RIGHT PARATRACHEAL LYMPH NODE". THERE ARE TWO PIECES OF RED AND
BLACK TISSUE INDIVIDUALLY MEASURING UP TO 0.6 CM IN GREATEST DIMENSION. ALL
EMBEDDED.

FROZEN SECTION DIAGNOSIS: NEGATIVE FOR NEOPLASM.

3. LABELLED "MEDIASTINAL LYMPH NODES X 3". THERE ARE FIVE PIECES OF SOFT
YELLOW AND TAN TISSUE MEASURING UP TO 0.6 CM IN GREATEST DIMENSION. MOST OF
THE TISSUE HAS THE APPEARANCE OF ADIPOSE TISSUE. WITHIN IT ARE TWO TAN AND
BLACK LYMPH NODES MEASURING 0.2 CM AND 0.5 CM IN GREATEST DIMENSION
RESPECTIVELY. THEY ARE BOTH ENTIRELY SUBMITTED FOR SECTIONING.   KAC/LMF

NAME: S.   M.   CONTINUED NEXTPAGE...   PATH #:   W-91-05099

KENNETH A. CLARK, M.D.
EDWARD D. MCDADE, M.D.

Winter Park Memorial Hospital
200 NORTH LAKEMONT AVENUE
WINTER PARK, FLORIDA 32792
(407) 646-7030

PATHOLOGIST CONSULTATION

NAME: S M   ROOM: ICU /ICU   PATH #:

HOSP#:   AGE: 70 YRS DOB: /21   SEX: M RACE: WHITE

DATE TAKEN: 09/24/91   DATE RECV'D: 09/25/91   DATE REPT: 09/25/91

PHYSICIAN: ROBINSON, HUGH B.   SURGEON: ROBINSON, HUGH

MACROSCOPIC DESCRIPTION:
----

4. LABELLED "RIGHT UPPER LOBE NODULE". THE SPECIMEN IS RECEIVED WITHOUT
FIXATIVE. THERE IS A WEDGE BIOPSY OF LUNG MEASURING 3.8 X 2.6 X 1.3 CM. ITS
EDGES CONTAIN ROWS OF STEEL STAPLES. THE PLEURAL SURFACE HAS A BRIGHT RED
APPEARANCE WITH PROMINENT ANTHRACOTIC PIGMENT MARKING. IMMEDIATELY BENEATH
THE PLEURA IS A 0.9 CM DIAMETER POORLY CIRCUMSCRIBED, SOFT TAN NODULE. IT
HAS VARIEGATED AREAS OF BLACK MARKING. THE ADJACENT LUNG PARENCHYMA HAS A
LIGHT RED AERATED APPEARANCE. REPRESENTATIVE SECTIONS ARE TAKEN.

FROZEN SECTION DIAGNOSIS: INFILTRATIVE ADENOCARCINOMA.   KAC/LMF

MICROSCOPIC DESCRIPTION:
----

1. PIECES OF LYMPH NODE ARE BLACKENED BY ANTHRACOTIC PIGMENT. NO NEOPLASM IS
SEEN. 88304,88331

2. TWO LYMPH NODES ARE BLACKENED BY ANTHRACOTIC PIGMENT. NO NEOPLASM IS
SEEN. 88304,88331

3. TWO LYMPH NODES ARE BLACKENED BY ANTHRACOTIC PIGMENT. NO NEOPLASM IS
SEEN. 88304,88331

4. LUNG PARENCHYMA CONTAINS A NODULAR AREA OF INFILTRATIVE MODERATELY
DIFFERENTIATED ADENOCARCINOMA. NEOPLASM EXTENDS EXTREMELY CLOSE TO THE
PLEURAL SURFACE. THE SURROUNDING LUNG PARENCHYMA IS UNREMARKABLE.
88305,88331   KAC/LMF

NAME: S   M   PATH #:   W-91-05099

FLORIDA HOSPITAL
Radiology Consultation

ORLANDO	(407) 897-1944	APOPKA	889-1059
OUTPATIENT CENTER	897-1565	ALTAMONTE	767-2208

FLORIDA RADIOLOGY ASSOCIATES, PA

PROBLEM: SYNCOPAL EPISODE.

PA AND LATERAL CHEST: 7/25/91

PA and lateral views show an unremarkable appearance of the heart and lungs. Degenerative changes are noted of the thoracic spine.

IMPRESSION: ESSENTIALLY NEGATIVE CHEST.

a gross misdiagnosis

✓

DAVID L. HOLDER, M.D./bc/7052

07/26/91 10:18:37

38-81-88   S   ,M
70 (DO   /21)
7/25/91   ALT/ER
CHEST PA AND LATERAL   JOHNSON, LESTER M.D.
                    Florida Hospital
               Altamonte Springs, Florida
                    Original   7251125.R1
              RADIOLOGY CONSULTATION

L: FB;DF

FLORIDA HOSPITAL
Radiology Consultation

ORLANDO	(407) 897-1944	APOPKA	889-1059
OUTPATIENT CENTER	897-1565	ALTAMONTE	767-2208

FLORIDA RADIOLOGY ASSOCIATES, PA

PROBLEM:`   CARDIOVASCULAR SYMPTOMS

OUTSIDE FILMS: 8-14-91

The outside film from Dr. West's office dated 12-28-90, has been   -
obtained and compared to the present film dated 7-25-91. The heart size
is stable. Lungs show a parenchymal nodule in the right mid lung which
appears probably diffusely calcified and is unchanged since the 12-90
film. *a missed diagnosis*

IMPRESSION: PARENCHYMAL NODULE ON THE RIGHT BETWEEN THE THIRD
                       AND FOURTH ANTERIOR RIBS WHICH IS UNCHANGED SINCE
                       PREVIOUS EXAMINATION. I SUSPECT THIS IS A
                       GRANULOMA. IF OLD FILMS ARE AVAILABLE TO FURTHER
                       COMPARE WITH THIS WOULD BE HELPFUL. IF NOT, THEN
                       FOLLOW UP FILM IN THREE MONTHS IS SUGGESTED.

CLIFFORD D. BIDWELL, M.D./EB

08/15/91 13:12:29

38-81-88	S M
70 (21)	
8-14-91	APOPKA/OP
OUTSIDE FILMS	WEST, H.K. ,M.D.

                            Florida Hospital
                            Apopka, Florida
                                Original   Remote Copy 1-2   814788.R1
                        RADIOLOGY CONSULTATION

L: FB;DB-2;AJ

FLORIDA HOSPITAL
Radiology Consultation

ORLANDO	(407) 897-1944	APOPKA	889-1059
OUTPATIENT CENTER	897-1565	ALTAMONTE	767-2208

FLORIDA RADIOLOGY ASSOCIATES, PA

PROBLEM: RIGHT SIDED NODULE.

COMPUTER TOMOGRAPHY SCAN OF THE CHEST: 8/20/91

Multiple axial images of the chest were obtained without contrast infusion and correlated with a chest film of 7/25/91. That film demonstrates a nodular opacity in peripheral aspect of right mid lung.

The CT images demonstrate no infiltrates. The nodule seen on chest x-ray is in the peripheral lateral aspect of the left upper lobe. Its contours are somewhat irregular. It is of soft tissue density.

There is an enlarged lymph node posterior to the ascending thoracic aorta of uncertain significance. No other enlarged mediastinal nodes are seen. Hila appear normal. Nodule in right upper lobe measures approximately 6 by 6 millimeter.

IMPRESSION: 1.   6 MILLIMETER NODULE IN PERIPHERAL LATERAL
                      ASPECT OF RIGHT UPPER LOBE. IT IS CONSISTENT
                      WITH BRONCHOGENIC CARCINOMA, METASTATIC LESION
                      OR GRANULOMA. COMPARISON WITH FILMS OLDER THAN
                      7/25/91 WOULD BE HELPFUL. FURTHER WORK UP IS
                      RECOMMENDED.

                2.   MILDLY ENLARGED MEDIASTINAL LYMPH NODE. THIS
                      COULD REPRESENT METASTATIC DISEASE OR POST
                      INFLAMMATORY CHANGE.

JAMES E. HANNAH, M.D./kmgg/0162

08/20/91   16:11:58

38-81-88
70 (··· , /21)   S.   , K
8/20/91   OP/ALT
CT CHEST   WEST, HAROLD KEN M.D./886-1300
                        Florida Hospital
                     Altamonte Springs, Florida
                            Original   820676.R1
                   RADIOLOGY CONSULTATION

L: FB;AJ

```
                                                                    RA
   ORLANDO, FL                                               13.17 09
                          ***     RADIOLOGY     ***
                       * *    I N T E R I M   R E P O R T        * *

   - - - - - - - - - - - - - - - - - - - - - - - - - - - - - - - - - - -
   PATIENT: 62955    S.        .M. RTO           MRI: 0388188
   EXAM:      BRAIN CT W&WO CONT.      70470  EXAM NUMBER: 9124900371
   EXAM TIME: 10:41                              FINAL
   - - - - - - - - - - - - - - - - - - - - - - - - - - - - - - - - - - -

   PROBLEM:        R/O METS

   ***** CLERICAL REVISION *****


   CT SCAN OF THE BRAIN:              9/6/91


   SCANNING WAS PERFORMED BEFORE AND FOLLOWING 100 CC OF ISOVUE INJECTED
   INTRAVENOUSLY.   MILD PATCHY CORTICAL ATROPHY IS PRESENT.  NO FOCAL
   MASSES. MASS EFFECT OR ENHANCING LESIONS ARE IDENTIFIED.


   IMPRESSIONS:        ATROPHY. NO ACUTE DISEASE.




   FENTON E. FROOM, M.D./JP/6377




   - - - - - - - - - - - - - - - - - - - - - - - - - - - - - - - - - - -
   RADIOLOGIST: FROOM,FENTON E.   MD          TRANSCRIPTIONIST  RT19
                                                        R609-R9
```

ORLANDO, FL   13.15 09/13

```
                    ***   RADIOLOGY      ***
                *  *  I N T E R I M   R E P O R T        *  *
- - - - - - - - - - - - - - - - - - - - - - - - - - - - - - - - - - - - - - - - -
PATIENT:  625.       S      .M                  MRI: 0388188
EXAM:     BONE SCAN              78306  EXAM NUMBER: 9124900373
EXAM TIME: 13:44                               FINAL
- - - - - - - - - - - - - - - - - - - - - - - - - - - - - - - - - - - - - - - - -

PROBLEM:           R/O LUNG CANCER



ISOTOPE BONE SCAN:                 09/06/91
```

25 MCI OF TECHNETIUM 99 M MDP WAS INJECTED INTRAVENOUSLY AND ROUTINE-
FRONTAL AND POSTERIOR VIEWS OBTAINED. THERE IS A MODERATE FOCAL
INCREASE IN ACTIVITY IN THE REGION OF THE RIGHT HIP. IT IS DIFFICULT TO
SAY WHETHER IT IS ACTUALLY IN THE FEMORAL HEAD OR IN THE ACETABULUM
ITSELF. PLAIN FILMS OF THE RIGHT HIP ARE RECOMMENDED FOR FURTHER
EVALUATION. IT IS SUSPICIOUS FOR METASTATIC DISEASE PARTICULARLY
CONSIDERING THE HISTORY.

INCREASE IN ACTIVITY IS NOTED IN THE RIGHT SHOULDER. PERHAPS MORE LIKELY
IN THE ACROMION. PLAIN FILMS OF THE RIGHT SHOULDER ARE RECOMMENDED FOR
FURTHER EVALUATION.

THERE ARE A FEW OTHER PERIPHERAL JOINT CHANGES PARTICULARLY IN THE LEFT
KNEE AND ANKLE CONSISTENT WITH OSTEOARTHRITIS. THE CENTRAL SPINE IS
INTACT.

BILATERAL RENAL EXCRETION OCCURS.

CONTINUED ON NEXT PAGE......

CONTINUED.........

- -
RADIOLOGIST: FROOM.FENTON E. MD   TRANSCRIPTIONIST: RT19
                                                    R609-R97
```
```

```
                                                                                RR770?
  ORLANDO, FL                                                            13.18 09/10/

                        ***     RADIOLOGY      ***
                   * *    I N T E R I M   R E P O R T        * *

 - - - - - - - - - - - - - - - - - - - - - - - - - - - - - - - - - - - - - - -
  PATIENT: 629F-      S'       '.M' ' ' '            MRI: 0388188
  EXAM:      BONE SCAN            78306  EXAM NUMBER: 9124900373
  EXAM TIME: 13:44                               FINAL
 - - - - - - - - - - - - - - - - - - - - - - - - - - - - - - - - - - - - - - -



  IMPRESSIONS:          ABNORMAL ACTIVITY OF THE RIGHT HIP AND RIGHT
                        SHOULDER SUGGESTING METASTATIC DISEASE BUT PLAIN
                        FILMS ARE RECOMMENDED FOR COMPARISON.




  FENTON E. FROOM, M.D./JP/6377
```

```
 - - - - - - - - - - - - - - - - - - - - - - - - - - - - - - - - - - - - - -
  RADIOLOGIST: FROOM,FENTON E.    MD              TRANSCRIPTIONIST: RT19
                                                             R609-R97?
```

```
   . .                    *** RADIOLOGY     ***
                     * *  I N T E R I M   R E P O R T    * *

 -- -- -- --  -- -- -- --  -- -- -- --  -- -- -- --  -- -- -- --  -- -- --
 PATIENT:          S       ,M         MRI: 0388188
 EXAM:     ABD CT W&W/O CONT.     74170  EXAM NUMBER: 9124900370
 EXAM TIME: 10:41                        FINAL
 -- -- -- --  -- -- -- --  -- -- -- --  -- -- -- --  -- -- -- --  -- -- --


 PROBLEM:          R/O METS


 ***** CLERICAL REVISION *****

 CT SCAN OF THE ABDOMEN:    9/6/91



 SCANNING WAS PERFORMED BEFORE AND FOLLOWING 100 CC OF ISOVUE INJECTED
 INTRAVENOUSLY.   ORAL CONTRAST WAS ALSO ADMINISTERED.

 THERE ARE ABOUT 4 LESIONS IN THE UPPER RIGHT LOBE OF THE LIVER.  THEY
 ARE LOWER IN ATTENTUATION THAN NORMAL LIVER BEFORE AND FOLLOWING IV
 CONTRAST.  AN ULTRASOUND EXAMINATION IS RECOMMENDED FOR FURTHER
 EVALUATION.  THEY MAY BE JUST CYSTS SINCE THEY ARE FAIRLY WELL
 CIRCUMSCRIBED BUT SUBTLE METASTATIC DEPOSITS CANNOT TOTALLY BE EXCLUDED.
 ONE OR TWO OF THESE MIGHT EVEN BE A HEMANGIOMA SINCE FOLLOWING CONTRAST
 THE EDGE OF ONE MAY BE FILLED IN SLIGHTLY OR THIS COULD JUST BE A
 PARTIAL VOLUME LOSS.  THE LOWER PORTION OF THE LIVER IS INTACT.

 THERE IS A ROUND ENLARGEMENT OF THE RIGHT ADRENAL GLAND UP TO 2 CM IN
 DIAMETER.  THERE IS ALSO WHAT APPEARS TO BE DIFFUSE ENLARGEMENT OF THE
 LEFT ADRENAL BUT IT IS STILL SOMEWHAT Y SHAPED.  BOTH THESE FINDINGS ARE
 SUSPICIOUS FOR METASTATIC DISEASE.  THERE IS A MASS IN WHAT MAY BE THE
 CEPHALAD PORTION OF THE HEAD OF THE PANCREAS OR IT IS A MASS OR
 ADENOPATHY JUST ADJACENT TO THE HEAD.  THE MASS MEASURES ABOUT 4.5 CM IN
 ITS GREATEST DIAMETER AND HAS IRREGULAR PERIPHERAL AND PARTIAL CENTRAL
 ENHANCEMENT FOLLOWING IV CONTRAST.  IT IS ESSENTIALLY A MASS LYING IN
 THE PORTAHEPATUS.  WITH THE HISTORY GIVEN IT IS ALSO SUSPICIOUS FOR
 METASTATIC DISEASE.


 CONTINUED ON NEXT PAGE......


 CONTINUED.........




 -- -- -- --  -- -- -- --  -- -- -- --  -- -- -- --  -- -- -- --  -- -- --
 RADIOLOGIST: FROOM,FENTON E.  MD           TRANSCRIPTIONIST: RT19
                                                          R609-RS
```

```
  ORLANDO, FL                      ***   RADIOLOGY   ***                    13.17 05
                          * *   I N T E R I M   R E P O R T         * *

  - -  -  -  - - - - - - - -  -  - -  -  - - - - - - - -  - -  -  -  -  - -  -
  PATIENT:   _        S░░░░, .M░░░░              MRI: 0388188
  EXAM:      ABD CT W&W/O CONT.        74170   EXAM NUMBER: 9124900370
  EXAM TIME: 10:41                             FINAL
  - -  -  -  - - - - - - - -  -  - -  -  - - - - - - - -  - -  -  -  -  - -  -
```

NO OTHER RETROPERITONEAL MASS OR ADENOPATHY IS SEEN.

IMPRESSIONS: AT LEAST FOUR LIVER LESIONS. RECOMMEND
                      ULTRASONOGRAPHY FOR FURTHER EVALUATION.

                      4.5 MASS IN THE PORTAHEPATUS OR UPPER PANCREATIC
                      HEAD.

                      ENLARGEMENT OF BOTH ADRENAL GLANDS THIS IS
                      SUSPICIOUS FOR METASTATIC DISEASE.

FENTON E. FROOM, M.D./JP/6377

```
  - - -  - -  -  - - -  -  - - - - -  -  - -  - -  - - -  -  - - -  - -  - -
  RADIOLOGIST: FROOM,FENTON E.   MD                 TRANSCRIPTIONIST: RT19
                                                             R609-R9
```

WINTER PARK MEMORIAL HOSPITAL
WINTER PARK, FLORIDA
RADIOLOGY REPORT

DATE: __9-24-91_____   X-Ray No. __1163745_____

PA AND LATERAL CHEST:

The lungs are well expanded. There are no effusions or acute infiltrates.
Pulmonary nodule seen in the right lung laterally as seen by computed
tomographic scan from outside hospital. Cardiovascular structures are
unremarkable. Osseous structures demonstrate degenerative changes.

IMPRESSION:

Right pulmonary nodule. No acute superimposed disease is noted.

Donal~~dor~~ ~~Bye~~ ~~Boddaa~~rd, M.D./mpk   PAGE 1 of 1
D:9-24/T:9-24-1991
Printed on 9-24-1991 10:23:14 A

1-5 (Rev. 4/89)

PHYSICIAN'S COPY

S ....., M.	
Patient Name	
230728	TBAS-1
Hospital No.	Room No.
Hugh B. Robinson, M.D.	
Physician	

FLORIDA HOSPITAL MEDICAL CENTER   DC979C0H
FL HOSPITAL, ORLANDO   15.37 02/09/93
                         RADIOLOGY
           * * *   F I N A L   R E P O R T   * * *

PATN ACCT: SC   , M   PATIENT MRI : .
EXAM DESC: CT ABDOMEN W&WO CONT   REQUIS NUMBER: 930359050100
EXAM DATE: 02/04/93   TRANS DATE: 02/04/93   RESULT STATUS: FIN

                        TRANS TIME: 16:53   REVISION NUM : 01

PROBLEM: NEOPLASM LUNG

COMPUTER TOMOGRAPHY SCAN OF ABDOMEN FOLLOWING ORAL CONTRAST MATERIAL
AND WITH AND WITHOUT INTRAVENOUS CONTRAST MATERIAL:

THERE ARE ONE, POSSIBLY TWO LESIONS NEAR THE DOME OF THE LIVER
POSTERIORLY. A THIRD LESION IS SEEN FURTHER CAUDALLY IN THE RIGHT LOBE
LATERALLY. A FIFTH LESION IS PROBABLY PRESENT IN THE CAUDATE LOBE. IN
ADDITION, THERE IS A LARGE MASS IN THE REGION OF THE PORTA HEPATIS AND
PERIPANCREATIC MASS. THE LARGE MASS COULD BE EASILY MEASURED AND IS 55
X 45 MM. THERE IS NO INTRAPERITONEAL FLUID. BOTH KIDNEYS ARE
FUNCTIONING. THE SPLEEN IS UNREMARKABLE. THERE ARE BILATERAL ADRENAL
MASSES.

IMPRESSION: THE PREVIOUS STUDY OF 09/10/91 HAS BEEN CHECKED OUT AND
               IS NOT AVAILABLE. THE PATIENT HAS A HISTORY OF CA OF THE
               LUNG.

               THERE ARE LIVER LESIONS, PORTAL AND PERIPANCREATIC LYMPH
               NODES THAT ARE ENLARGED AND BILATERAL ADRENAL MASSES, ALL
               CONSISTENT WITH METASTATIC DISEASE. AS FAR AS I CAN TELL
               FROM THE PREVIOUS REPORT, ALL THESE LESIONS WERE
               IDENTIFIED BEFORE.

CHARLES E. WALBROEL, MD/SM/5101

READING PHYSICIAN : DR CHARLES E. WALBROEL MD
ORDERING PHYSICIAN : DR PATRICIO P. GONZALES MD - (407)352-9717
SEX: M AGE: 71 Y (DOB 06/09/1921)   R888-R972
OUTPATIENT   TRANSCRIPTIONIST: RT6

                                              TOTAL P.01

20. Patient FA

DOB: 6/9/32

Patient FA is a 62 year-old white woman from Texas who in 1985 first developed digestive problems. Over the following years, her symptoms gradually worsened, and during 1989, she suffered chronic diarrhea, malaise and a 25-pound weight loss. In late September of 1989, she reports onset of severe abdominal pain, associated with worsening diarrhea. Her local physician referred her for an abdominal ultrasound that revealed a possible mass in the head of the pancreas. A CT scan of the abdomen confirmed the mass effect. ERCP performed September 9, 1989 demonstrated narrowing of the pancreatic duct traversing the pancreatic head (3 mm.) as compared to a 6 mm. duct traversing the body of the pancreas. With an uncertain diagnosis, she was placed on oral pancreatic enzymes for two weeks, with initial improvement in her symptoms followed by relapse. A repeat CT of the abdomen on October 13, 1989 again revealed a mass in the head of the pancreas, which was thought to be unchanged or possibly enlarged since the previous study one month earlier.

Patient FA was told she most likely had pancreatic cancer that required immediate surgery. However, when her doctors admitted surgery would not be curative, she decided to refuse all further intervention. Instead, Patient FA chose to pursue my protocol, and came to my office for her initial visit on November 2, 1989. At that time, she reported midabdominal pain radiating into her back, associated with chronic low-grade fevers and frequent sweats. She was taking Ogen 0.25 mg per day, Xanax TID, Fiorinal and Darvocet PRN. She denied any history of alcohol abuse. Her physical examination was unremarkable. CEA (Roche) drawn November 11, 1989 was 5.3.

Shortly after her visit to New York, Patient FA began her nutritional protocol that she has continued enthusiastically to the present time. On her protocol, she gained 40 pounds, says she is in the best health she has every known, denies any abdominal symptoms whatsoever and generally feels "wonderful."

After Patient FA had completed two years on her nutritional protocol, a repeat CT scan on November 4, 1991 was completely clear, with no evidence of the tumor.

I realize Patient FA is not a definitive case because of the lack of tissue diagnosis, but I think she has an interesting history, and illustrates how well the program works for pancreatic tumors.

Dr. Gonzalez presented these 25 cancer case studies to the NCI in 1993 and then updated the patient status information in 2001. Below are Dr. Gonzalez's personal notes with updated survival information:

Inoperable pancreatic cancer. Alive and well 11 years out. This patient's survival status was updated again in 2016. Please refer to page 257 for this additional information.

CENTRAL TEXAS MEDICAL CENTEF
P.O. BOX 767
SAN MARCOS, TEXAS 78667
512-353-6520

X-RAY REPORT

Family Name	First Name	Middle Name	Room No.	Patient No.
			OP	

Attending Physician		Date	Med. Rec. No.	Sex	Age	X-Ray No.
RICE		10-13-89	51724	F	57	6810

Report:

CT SCAN OF ABDOMEN:

A CT scan of the abdomen with both oral and IV contrast enhancement again reveals the mass effect in the region of the head of the pancreas. The low density area is at least the same size and may have actually increased minimally in size since the previous exam. No decrease in size of the mass effect is seen.

IMPRESSION:

No real appreciable change in the appearance of the CT of the pancreatic region since the previous exam. There has certainly been no decrease in size of the mass.

VAN E. REA, M.D./CWB/10-13-89

Signature of Roentgenologist

X-I
R
R

X-RAY REPORT

CENTRAL TEXAS MEDICAL CENTER
P.O. BOX 767
SAN MARCOS, TEXAS 78667
512-353-6520

Family Name	First Name	Middle Name		Room No.		Patient No.
F. A.				SGY		

Attending Physician			Date	Med. Rec. No.	Sex	Age	X-Ray No.
RICE			09-29-89	51724	F	57	6810

Report:

ERCP:

The pancreatic duct and common bile duct were opacified by Dr. Rice.
The cystic duct and gallbladder also opacify. No stones are
identified. The cystic duct is patent. The portion of the
pancreatic duct which traverses the pancreatic head is somewhat
narrowed and there is the suggestion of extrinsic pressure. This
narrowed portion of the duct measures approximately 3 mm in caliber.
The portion of the duct that traverses the body of the pancreas is
approximately 6 mm in caliber. The common bile duct measures a
maximum of 14 mm in caliber. Exam is otherwise unremarkable.

WILLIAM H. HEALY, M.D./CWB/09-29-89

_____
Signature of Roentgenologist

RADIOLOGY SERVICES - OUTPATIENT EXAMS

DATE EXAM	PHYSICIAN REQUESTING:	
11-4-91	RICE	

EXAMINATION REQUESTED:
CT ABD 5 MM CUTS PANCREAS

CLINICAL HISTORY / INDICATION FOR EXAMINATION:
PANCREATIC CANCER

PREVIOUS STUDY: YES ☐   NO ☐

WHERE?
SPECIAL INSTRUCTIONS:

ALLERGIES:

LMP:

CALL REPORT ☐   STAT READING ☐

IMPRINT AREA

91594600   RAD

6-9-32

CONTRAST	Hypaque	BUN	13
AMOUNT	150ml	CREAT.	1.0
	Power Inj yes	TIME RECEIVED	

TECH PERFORMING & COMMENTS:

TIME EXAM STARTED 0825
TIME EXAM COMPLETED 0915

Pt. SHIELDED
NO ☐   YES ☐

FILMS USED 26/c   REPEAT   07-90-97

RC

RADIOLOGY CONSULTATION

ABDOMINAL CT WITH THIN SECTION CUTS THROUGH THE PANCREAS   11-4-91   0915

Initial images were obtained through the upper abdomen including the pancreas following intravenous and oral contrast. Following pancreatic localization, 5mm thin section cuts are repeated through the pancreas.

Liver and spleen appear normal. The pancreas is well visualized and has a normal configuration with no evidence of pancreatic mass, peripancreatic infiltration, or abnormal pancreatic duct dilatation. Surrounding peripancreatic structures appear normal. Both adrenal glands, kidneys, and contrast filled bowel loops appear unremarkable.

CONCLUSIONS:

1   Normal abdominal CT with thin section images through the pancreas.

11-4-91/bf
1450

M. B. Martin, M.D.

DATE   RADIOLOGIST

SAMC-1206 (REV 11-89) ITEM # 725

Prostate Cancer

21. Patient MC
DOB:5/3/22

Patient MC is a 71 year-old white male with prostate cancer. In April of 1987, during a routine physical exam, he was found to have an enlarged hard prostate. Needle biopsy on May 5, 1987 revealed well-to-moderately differentiated infiltrating adenocarcinoma. A CT scan on May 20, 1987 demonstrated a significantly enlarged prostate, with no evidence of intra- or retroperitoneal masses. Patient MC was told that because the disease appeared to have spread outside the capsule, radiation, and not surgery, was the appropriate treatment. Patient MC, however, who had previously been on an aggressive nutritional program during the 1970's, refused all standard treatment.

He was first seen in my office on November 12, 1987. He denied voiding symptoms, but did report some fatigue and flare-up of bursitis. He was on no medications, and his examination was notable only for a hard, enlarged prostate.

Patient MC began his nutritional program upon returning to California. Since then he has also been followed by his local urologist. On March 24, 1988, after he had completed six months on his program, an ultrasound evaluation of the prostate indicated a 1.2 by 0.9 cm. focal hypoechoic lesion in the right peripheral zone towards the base, consistent with malignancy. A year later, on April 26, 1989, a repeat prostate ultrasound documented significant reduction in the tumor: this time, the report describes a 0.3 cm minute hypoechoic nodule in the right base.

Patient MC has now completed 5.5 years on his nutritional protocol, remains very compliant and is in excellent health. He denies any urinary tract symptoms, and says he hasn't felt so good "in years."

Dr. Gonzalez presented these 25 cancer case studies to the NCI in 1993 and then updated the patient status information in 2001. Below are Dr. Gonzalez's personal notes with updated survival information:

Stage IV prostate cancer. Alive and well 13 years out.

HUMANA HOSPITAL - WEST HILLS LABORATORY

PHONE: (818) 884-7060

7300 MEDICAL CENTER DRIVE
CANOGA PARK, CALIFORNIA 91307

PATHOLOGICAL REPORT

PATHOLOGISTS
Samuel Kremen, M.D.
Gary N. Pesselnick, M.D.

Date of Procedure __5/5/87__

Name __MC_____ C_____ L_____
          Last Name   First   Middle

Room No. __OP__

Doctor __KUNIN_____ Age: __65__ Hosp. No. __301019-6__

Specimen Site __Prostate_____ Specimen No. __H 1367-87__

GROSS DESCRIPTION

The specimen consists of three (3) gray-tan needle biopy cores, ranging up to 1.6 cm in length. Totally submitted.

MICROSCOPIC DESCRIPTION:

Examination of multiple sections reveals adenocarcinoma, generally characterized by small infiltrating glandular structures. Focally, perineural invasion is noted. Occasional larger glandular structures form a cribriform pattern. The neoplastic epithelial cells show mildly hyperchromatic and irregular nuclei. The tumor is found in all three (3) biopsy cores.

DIAGNOSIS:

NEEDLE BIOPSY SEGMENTS OF PROSTATE GLAND SHOWING WELL TO MODERATELY DIFFERENTIATED INFILTRATING PROSTATIC ADENOCARCINOMA.

GNP/eo
5/6/87

_____ M.D.
Pathologist

(LAB 4) 30504-2503 (9/84)
0016599

202

Humana Hospital–West Hills
DEPARTMENT OF DIAGNOSTIC IMAGING
7300 Medical Center Dr. • Canoga Park, CA 91307
(818) 712-4119

RONALD YULISH, M.D.
IRVING B. RAYMAN, M.D.
RICHARD E. RUBENSTEIN, M.D.
MICHAEL M. LITWIN, M.D.

RICHARD M. GALINSON, M.D.
BRUCE A. SHRAGG, M.D.
ROBERT HOWARD, M.D.
GARY J. GOSS, M.D.
ROBERT A. PRINCENTHAL, M.D.

DIPLOMATES OF THE AMERICAN BOARD OF RADIOLOGY

OP

5/20/87   9:27AM X/R   CHARGE   001 R   00704857-2 5/20/87

M   C   L
000000011373 DOB: /22
ALIGN NEOPL PROSTATE   065 M KUNIN, SAMUEL
    ft   in   lbs   ozs ALLERGY :

26-86202 CT PELVIS W& W/O CONTRAST 721949   Item:86202   Qty :01

OP :X/R

REPORT   DATE OF EXAM: 5/20/87   X-RAY NO

CT OF THE PELVIS:

AP scoutviews were obtained for localization. Pre and post contrast enhanced
scans of the pelvis were obtained after ingestion of 150 cc of 2% Gastrografin.
The intravenous contrast agent used was 200 cc of Conray 43.
                    appeared
The prostate to be enlarged. No intra- or retropelvic masses were seen.
The bladder showed normal contours. There was no evidence of fluid in
the pelvis.

IMPRESSION:

SOMEWHAT ENLARGED PROSTATE. NO INTRA- OR RETROPELVIC MASSES WERE SEEN.

RMG/re   RICHARD M. GALINSON, M.D.

SCAN**UR** SERVICES
Mobile Urological Ultrasound

1640 Haynes Lane
Redondo Beach, CA 90278
(213) 372-0800

Patient: M   , C
Date of Examination: 3/24/88
Physician: Samuel A. Kunin, M.D.

ULTRASOUND EXAMINATION OF THE PROSTATE

PROCEDURE

A realtime ultrasound examination of the prostate was performed
with a transrectal biplane transducer. Images were recorded in
the axial and sagittal projections.

FINDINGS

There is moderate enlargement of the transition zone. The
appearance of the transition zone is consistent with BPH. The
volume of the gland corresponds to a weight of 37 grams.

The seminal vesicles are symmetric in appearance.

In the right peripheral zone towards the base an approximately
1.2 x .9 cm focal hypoechoic abnormality is noted. There are
calcifications within the gland most noted along the urethra.

The remainder of the parenchyma of the gland has a normal
ultrasound appearance and the capsule is intact.

Impressions

Abnormal transrectal prostate ultrasound demonstrating the
presence of a 1.2 x .9 cm focal hypoechoic change noted in the
right peripheral zone towards the base. This finding is
consistent when considered with the clinical history ~~and~~ with
malignancy.

By ultrasound staging this would be consistent with a UB 1
lesion. If clinically indicated, correlation of this focal
hypoechoic change with ultrasound directed biopsy is suggested.

Judith G. Rose, M.D.

TRANS-MEDICAL IMAGING
PORTABLE ULTRASOUND SERVICES

P.O. BOX 2111
THOUSAND OAKS, CA 91360-0918
805-492-1980

PT: M.   . C.   **DATE:** 4/26/89

AGE: 67   **SEX:** male   **PHYSICIAN:** Dr. Kunin

PROSTATE ULTRASOUND:

Examination was performed using the 7.5 MHz endorectal probe. Axial and sagittal views were performed. The prostate is moderately enlarged consistent with hyperplasia with scattered calcification in the surgical capsule consistent with corpora amylacea. Compared to previous exam done on 3/24/88, a faint minute hypoechoic nodule is seen in the right base measuring approximately 3 mm.'s in diameter. Nodule is not well-seen; however, the nodule has not grown in comparison to previous exam. No other hypoechoic nodules are seen.

CONCLUSION:

1. Minute 3 mm. faintly seen hypoechoic nodule seen in the right peripheral base.

JN:lam

J. Newton, M.D.

22. Patient RV
DOB 9/3/20

Patient RV is a 72 year-old white male with a history of widely metastatic prostate cancer. He had been in good health when a routine blood screen in March of 1990 revealed an elevated PSA and PAP (prostatic acid phosphatase) at 7.0 and 76.8 respectively. A needle biopsy of the prostate in April confirmed carcinoma, but both bone scan and CT of the abdomen were negative for metastatic disease.

In May of 1990, Patient RV began a course of radiation to the prostate and pelvis with curative intent, for what was considered stage B disease. After completion of radiotherapy, both PSA and PAP returned to normal levels. He subsequently did well for more than a year, except for recurrent radiation induced enteritis, until late August, 1991 when the PSA rose to 288 and the PAP increased to 494. A repeat bone scan on August 28, 1991 demonstrated extensive new osseous metastases of the total spine, thorax, and scapula, all consistent with metastatic disease. A CT scan of the pelvis August 27, 1991 showed extension of tumor beyond the prostatic capsule. Because of these findings, on September 25, 1991, Patient RV underwent bilateral orchiectomy at Providence Hospital, in Seattle, Washington. After surgery, he was seen at the University of Washington and initially entered into the SWOG protocol that was evaluating the postorchiectomy use of flutamide. However, Patient RV refused to take his medication because of possible side effects and dropped out of the study.

After surgery, Patient RV's PSA dropped to 156 on October 29, 1991. A follow-up CT scan of the cervical spine on September 11, 1991 documented blastic lesions involving the skull base and cervical spine. An MRI on November 23, 1991—two months after surgery—revealed extensive bony metastases throughout the spine from the cervical level to the sacrum.

However, throughout the fall of 1991, the PSA continued to drop, reaching 147 on November 27. Then in December 1991, Patient RV consulted Dr. Jonathan Collin, a nutritionally oriented physician in Washington State. Dr. Collin started the patient on an aggressive nutritional protocol, and the PSA continued to fall, reaching a low of 84.2 on January 27, 1992.

At that point, Dr. Collin referred Patient RV to me. I first saw him in my office on February 18, 1992. At that time, he denied any bone pain or urinary symptoms, and his physical examination was unremarkable.

On February 25, 1992, after returning to Seattle, he went for another PSA which came back elevated at 90.6—the first rise since his orchiectomy. Three days later, on February 28, Patient RV began his protocol. And, over the next nine months, his PSA gradually dropped, reaching 21.6 on November 30, 1992, the lowest level since immediately after radiotherapy in May 1990.

In January 1993, an abdominal ultrasound was negative. The most recent PSA test from March 1993 was somewhat elevated at 41.5: at that time, Patient RV had been off his protocol for several weeks because of recurrent gastroenteritis. However, he is again on his program and the PSA will be repeated shortly.

Patient RV has completed nearly 17 months on his nutritional protocol, and reports that he is in excellent health. I believe he is an interesting patient because of the steady PSA drop he experienced while on the program—and the slight elevation that occurred when he was temporarily off.

Dr. Gonzalez presented these 25 cancer case studies to the NCI in 1993 and then updated the patient status information in 2001. Below are Dr. Gonzalez's personal notes with updated survival information:

Stage IV prostate cancer. Quit the program after enjoying significant improvement after 2 years. Lost to follow-up.

PACIFIC MEDICAL CENTER

PHYSICIAN/SURGEON	SIGNATURE & TITLE	PHAMIS USER ID NO.	LOCATION (CLINIC, ROOM, WARD, ETC.)
Dr Gerber		17556	Urology MAY 90 -11 07

SPECIMEN

Prostate needle Bx X4

BRIEF CLINICAL HISTORY & OPERATIVE FINDINGS (INCLUDE DURATION OF LESION AND RAPIDITY OF GROWTH, IF A NEOPLASM)

*Send Report to Dr Wonderly
Abn. Prostate W/S R/O Prostate Ca*

PREOPERATIVE DIAGNOSIS

? Prostate Ca

POSTOPERATIVE DIAGNOSIS

DATE OBTAINED 5/3/90

PATHOLOGICAL REPORT

1393

GROSS

5/3/90 The specimen is received in four parts.

A: The specimen is received in formalin with the designation "prostate needle biopsy, site not specified." The specimen consists of two similar appearing, variously sized minute portions of pinkish-grey tissue, varying in size from less than 0.1 to 0.4 x less than 0.1 cm in width. The tissue is totally submitted.

B. The specimen is received in formalin with the designation "prostatic needle biopsy, site not specified." The specimen consists of a single cylindrical, pinkish-grey tissue measuring 0.7 x 0.1 cm in width. The tissue is totally submitted.

C. The specimen is received in formalin with the designation "prostatic needle biopsy, site not specified." The specimen consists of a single cylindrical pinkish-grey tissue measuring 1.0 x 0.1 cm in width. The tissue is totally submitted.

D. The specimen is received in formalin with the designation "prostatic needle biopsy, site not specified." The specimen consists of two tubular pinkish-grey tissues ranging in size from 0.5 x 0.1 to 0.6 by less than 0.1 cm in width. The tissue is totally submitted.

MICROSCOPIC

5/4/90 A. Sections reveal small portions of fibro muscular stroma containing nerve structures. There are no glandular structures seen in the sections examined.

B, C, and D. Sections reveal prostatic tissue containing a

PATHOLOGIST	DATE	ACCESSION NO.(S)
Alicia D. Buyco, MD.	5/7/90	S90-1393

PATHOLOGIST SIGNATURE

PT. ID.

70 44 70 08
L
25SEP20
532-12-7936 EXP 7SEP90
SSA

SUBMITTING FACILITY
- BEACON HILL 1200 12th Ave S, Seattle, WA 98144 326-4000
- TOTEM LAKE 13118 121st Wy N E, Kirkland, WA 98034 ... 823-8405
- RENTON 17800 Talbot Rd S, Renton, WA 98055...............255-4045
- NORTH 10416 5th Ave N E, Seattle, WA 98125................ 526-1509
- BELLEVUE 14730 N E 8th, Bellevue, WA 98007...............644-9533
- PROVIDENCE 1600 E Jefferson #315, Seattle, WA 98122...326-4075
- Other

PACIFIC MEDICAL CENTER
TISSUE EXAMINATION
PA-0018 (8/88)

malignant neoplasm, composed of proliferating disorganized neoplastic cells arranged as glandular structures, for the most part, separated by dense connective tissue stroma. In some areas glands are smaller and fused. Nuclei are large irregular, hyperchromatic or vesicular, many with prominent nucleoli, and the cytoplasm is scanty to fairly adequate and pale staining. Elsewhere, nerve structures show invasion of their perineural lymphatic spaces by tumor. In focal areas, chronic inflammatory cells are also observed.

DIAGNOSIS: A. "Prostatic needle biopsy, site not specified" showing portions of fibromuscular stroma with no evidence of malignancy.
B, C and D. "Prostatic needle biopsies, sites not specified" showing poorly differentiated adenocarcinoma, Gleason's pattern IV, with perineural lymphatic invasion.

PMC

PACIFIC MEDICAL CENTER AND CLINICS
1200 12th Ave. S., Seattle, WA 98144
(206) 326-4000 EXT. 2500

Clinical Laboratory Report

R' . , V '   AD MED   8/28
                                                                              07:4

          70447008   M   70   DUNNING, STEVE MD-PRIM C

<<<<<<<<<<<<<<<<<<<<<<<<<<<<<<<<<<<<< CHEMISTRY >>>>>>>>>>>>>>>>>>>>>>>>>>>>>>>>>>

              ACID PHS RIA
    SERUM   PAP   PSA
    NORMALS   0.0-3.2   0.0-4.0
    UNITS   NG/ML   NG/ML
 AUG 26 0920 494.0HT 1   288.0   HT
       (8/27/91)
       *1 CONFIRMED BY DILUTION METHOD. DR. TO BE CLLD IN AM 8-28-91

       PERMANENT COPY - FOR MEDICAL RECORDS
       R'   V.   70447008   AD MED   8/28

```
  PTH: 76447008  NAME: RUSPES, V....         SEX: M  DOB: 23Sep1
920                              PAGE: 1
ar93           DATES:    29Mar93      23Mar93      25Mar93      25M
02pm           TIME:     9:18am       2:30pm       4:03pm        4:

          SPEC   TEST
               LAST PREVIOUS  DATE

                                        HEMATOLOGY
          COMPLETE BLOOD COUNT            |        |         |
       B   WBC (K/UL)          4.06 l |- |        |         |
       B   RBC (M/UL)          4.41     |   .     |         |
       B   HGB (GM/DL)         13.8     |        |         |
       B   HCT (%)             40.1     |        |         |
       B   MCV (FL)            90.9     |        |         |
       B   MCH (PG)            31.3     |        |         |
       B   MCHC (%)            34.4     |        |         |
       B   RDW-CV (%)          14.0     |        |         |
       B   RDW-SD (FL)         46.5     |        |         |
       B   PLT (K/UL)          279.     |        |         |
       B   MPV (FL)            10.6     |        |         |
          DIFFERENTIAL                  |        |         |
       B   SEG (%)             55.      |        |         |
       B   LYMPH (%)           32.      |        |         |
       B   MONO (%)            5.       |        |         |
       B   EOSIN (%)           3.       |        |         |
       B   BASO (%)            2.       |        |         |
       B   ATY LYM             3.       |        |         |
       B   PLT EST             NORM     |        |         |
       B   MORPH               NORM     |        |         |

                                        MAIN CHEMISTRY
          ELECTROLYTES                  |        |         |
       S   NA (MEQ/L)          140.     | .      |         |
       S   K (MEQ/L)           4.3      |        |         |
       S   CL (MEQ/L)          106.     |        |         |
       S   CO2 (MEQ/L)         26.      |        |         |
          CHEM I                        |        |         |
       S   GLU (MG/DL)         89.      |        |         |
       S   BUN (MG/DL)         11.      |        |         |
       S   CREAT (MG/DL)       1.1      |   .    |         |
       S   URIC (MG/DL)        5.7      |        |         |
       S   CHOL (MG/DL)       (273.) h  |        |         |
       S   T BILI (MG/DL)      0.3      |        |         |
       S   D BILI (MG/DL)      0.1   .  |        |         |
       S   TP (G/DL)           6.4  l   |        |         |
       S   ALB (G/DL)          3.5      | .      |         |
       S   CA (MG/DL)          9.1      |        |         |
          ENZYMES                       |        |         |
       S   LDH (IU/L)          158.     |        |         |
       S   SGOT (IU/L)         23.      |        |         |
       S   SGPT (IU/L)         19.      |        |         |
       S   ALP (IU/L)          203.     |        |         |
       S   PSA (NG/ML)                  |  41.5 h |        |
```

DR GONZALEZ COPY

Page 1 of 1

Examination(s) Performed:	Facility:	Patient Location:
BONE IMAGING, WHOLE BODY	CENT	

Specific reason for this examination:
? METS.

History/Pertinent Clinical Findings:
PROSTATE CANCER.

Requesting Provider:	User Number:	Request Date:	Study Date:
WONDERLY, RICHARD	11736		15May1990

INTERPRETATION

BONE SCAN:

DOSE: 25 mCi Tc 99m MDP IV.

FINDINGS:

Three hour delayed images of the whole body, with multiple spot views
of the axial skeleton were obtained after IV injection of 25 mCi Tc
99m MDP. There is modest increased uptake associated with the right
AC joint and to a lesser extent the remainder of the right shoulder.
There is very minor increased uptake associated with both hips. No
focal abnormal increased or decreased uptake identified to suggest
metastatic disease. Renal uptake and excretion is unremarkable.

RESIDENT: Marcus Whitley, M.D.

Impression:

No evidence of metastatic disease.

ROBERT GRIEP, M.D./ RG
Date Authenticated: 22May1990

Dictated: 16May1990   Transcribed: 17May1990   Transcriptionist: CB

	Age: 69	Diagnostic Imaging Report
70447008		Nuclear Medicine
		Phone: (206) 326-4009
R~~~ , V		
J4 .23Sep1920	M	
PAT SSN:	[CENT]	
GUAR SSN:		

PACIFIC
MEDICAL CENTER

1200 12th Ave. S. Seattle, WA 98144

MR-0043 (REV 4/86)

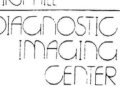

R‾ ^ _,_V‾ ‾
DOB: 9/23/20
6642

CT PELVIS WITH CONTRAST: 8/27/91

CLINICAL HISTORY:

Patient with previously diagnosed prostatic carcinoma. Evaluate for extracapsular extension.

TECHNIQUE:

Serial axial 10 mm scans were done from just above the iliac crest inferiorly to the superior acetabular region followed by contiguous 5 mm scans through the inferior pelvis to better evaluate the prostate. As the patient had a history of prior contrast reaction and in that there was a previous study for comparison (5-15-90) intravneous contrast was not given for today's study.

FINDINGS:

Comparison of today's study with that of 5-15-90 shows very little change in the appearance of either the seminal vesicles or prostate. There is some nodularity and stranding in the periprostatic plexus, but this is stable to slightly improved relative to the earlier scan and is not felt to represent periprostatic adenopathy. Some small phleboliths are seen in vessles along the left side of the prostate.

The contours of the prostate show slight asymmetric fullness along the right lateral superior aspect of the gland just below its junction with the seminal vesicles as can be seen on axial image 24 (2/4, 4/4). In addition, there is slight fullness along the mid to left posterior aspect of the gland below the midglandular level on image 27. This is a slight, subtle change in the glandular contour since May 15, 1990. Periprostatic fat is still evident adjacent to the right superolateral asymmetry while the fat plane between the rectum and the posterior margin of the prostate is blurred along that area of asymmetry in the posterior-inferior aspect of the gland.

No other abnormalities are seen through the extent of this scan.

IMPRESSION:

1. Slight asymmetry along the right superolateral margin of the gland near the glandular base and fullness and slight asymmetry along the posterior margin of the gland between the midglandular level and the apex.

(CONTINUED)

1001 Boylston Avenue   Seattle, Washington 98104   206/329-MRMR (6767)   FAX# 206/323-6989

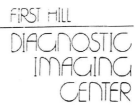

R   , V
DOB: 9/23/20
6642

CT PELVIS WITH CONTRAST: 8/27/91

(CONTINUED - PAGE 2)

Both of these are subtle, but are felt to be new findings relative
to 5-15-90. As such, they are suspicious for but not diagnostic
for capsular and immediate paracapsular extension of tumor.
However, this must be correlated with the results of biopsy
specimens and the known distribution of tumor in this patient as
other conditions, such as prostatitis, might also result in such
changes. There is no gross extension of tumor to pelvic sidewalls
or to immediate periprostatic structures.

2. No other abnormalities defined.

JWB:glh
Referring Physician:
RICHARD K. WONDERLY, M.D.

JAMES W. BORROW, M.D.

1001 Boylston Avenue   Seattle, Washington 98104   206/329-MRMR (6767)   FAX# 206/323-6989

Page 1 of 1

Examination(s) Performed:	Facility:	Patient Location:
CERVICAL SPINE 4 VIEWS	BHILL	PC

Specific reason for this examination:
EVALUATE FOR METS.

History/Pertinent Clinical Findings:
BONE SCAN SHOWS AREAS CONSISTENT WITH METS IN CERVICAL SPINE,
LUMBAR SPINE AND RIBS. PROSTATE CA W/ELEVATED PSA.

Requesting Provider:	User Number:	Request Date:	Study Date:
DUNNING, STEVE	8113	28Aug1991	28Aug1991

INTERPRETATION

CERVICAL, THORACIC AND LUMBOSACRAL SPINE:

The thoracic and lumbosacral spine show no visible changes since the examination of 10 June '91 and 15 February '98. Specifically, I see no changes suggestive of metastatic disease.

In the cervical spine, there are no comparison films. There is a sclerotic lesion of the dorsal spine of C4 which is probably a metastatic deposit. No other metastases are demonstrated by this study.

The absence of radiographic changes in the face of a positive bone scan makes metastatic disease almost a certainty. Bone scan changes often lead radiographic changes by weeks to months.

Impression:

1. Metastatic deposit in C4.
2. Negative thoracic and lumbar spine.

FREDERIC H. GERBER, M.D./ FG
Date Authenticated: 29Aug1991

Dictated: 28Aug1991	Transcribed: 29Aug1991	Transcriptionist: CB

70447008	Age: 70	Diagnostic Imaging Report
, V.		Radiology
		Phone: (206) 326-4123
J4 23Sep1920	M	
PAT SSN:	[BHILL]	
GUAR SSN:		

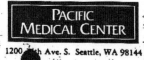

PACIFIC MEDICAL CENTER
1200 th Ave. S. Seattle, WA 98144

XR-0043 (R5-91)

Examination(s) Performed: Facility: Patient Location:
  BONE/JOINT IMAGING,WHOLE BODY   BHILL   PC

Specific reason for this examination:
  INCREASED PSA, CARCINOMA OF THE PROSTATE.

History/Pertinent Clinical Findings:

  185

Requesting Provider: User Number: Request Date: Study Date:
  DUNNING, STEVE   8113   28Aug1991

I N T E R P R E T A T I O N

TOTAL BODY BONE SCAN:

DOSE: 25 mCi Tc 99m MDP

REPORT:

Comparison bone scan is dated 15May90. Following intraveneous
administration of the radiopharmaceutical, delayed anterior and
posterior images of the skeleton were acquired. Compared to 14May90,
there are multiple abnormal foci of increased activity, these include
the base of the skull, C4, C5, and C6 vertebral bodies, T3, T8, and
T11 vertebral bodies, the posterior elements of T2, T6, and T7, L2
vertebral body, the posterior elements of L1, L3, and L4, the left
posterior ribs one, five, six, seven, eight, and eleven, the anterior
left two, five, and eighth ribs, the lateral six, seven, and tenth
ribs, the right posterior seventh rib, the right anterior two, four,
six, seven, and eighth ribs, the right lateral eighth and ninth ribs,
the right scapular tip, the left scapular spine and the sternum.
There are no lesions involving the pelvis or distal extremities.

IMPRESSION:

Interval development of extensive osseous metastases of the total
spine, thorax, and scapula. Plain radiographs of the spine are
recommended to further evaluate these areas. The patient's physician,
Dr. Dunning was notified.

RESIDENT: Sharon K. Wallace, M.D.

	Age: 70	Diagnostic Imaging Report
70447008		Nuclear Medicine
		Phone: (206) 326-4009
R , V		
J4 23Sep1920	M	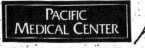
	[BHILL]	PACIFIC MEDICAL CENTER
PAT SSN:		1200 12th Ave. S. Seattle, WA 98144
GUAR SSN:		XR-0043 (R5-91)

R ⌐) **V** ...

DOB: 9/23/20
6642

CT OF THE CERVICAL SPINE WITHOUT CONTRAST::   9/11/91

DIAGROSTIC
IMAGING
CENTER

CLINICAL HISTORY:

70 year old man whose 8-28-91 bone scan is said to have shown
multiple abnormalities involving the skull base and cervical
spine from C4 through C6. Evaluate for extent of disease to help
plan radiation therapy.

TECHNIQUE:

Using contiguous 4 mm sections, the cervical spine was scanned
from the skull base through T1. The examination is reviewed with
the 8-28-91 bone scan from Pacific Medical Center.

FINDINGS:

A number of abnormally-sclerotic areas are identified within the
trabecular bone but these do not distort the cortex and none of
the lesions compromises the spinal canal. Sclerotic lesions
involve the left occipital bone at the level of the foramen magnum
(image C3), the right pedicle of C4 (image C20), the right pedicle
of C5 (image C24), and the spinous process of C7 (C34 - C35).

Mild degenerative disc disease leads to flattening of the anterior
thecal sac at C3-C4 and mild narrowing of the neural foramina at
C3-C4 and C6-C7.

IMPRESSION:

1. Sclerotic lesions, consistent with blastic metastases of
prostate carcinoma involve the skull base and cervical spine as
described above. The lesions do not compromise the spinal canal.

2. Mild degenerative disc disease at C3-C4 and C6-C7.

JPS:glh
Referring Physician:
MEHMET FER, M.D.

JUSTIN P. SMITH, M.D.

1001 Boylston Avenue   Seattle. Washington 98104   206/329-MRMR (6767)   FAX# 206/323-6989

R░░ ░3, V░░░
DOB: 09/23/20
SEX: M
6642 *70 44 70 08*

MR OF THE CERVICAL, THORACIC & LUMBAR SPINE: 11/21/91

CLINICAL HISTORY:
Patient with bony metastatic disease secondary to prostatic
carcinoma. Now with lower extremity numbness. Evaluate for cord-
and nerve root-compromising lesions.

TECHNIQUE:
Sagittal T1-weighted spin-echo sequences of the cervical,
thoracic and lumbar spine with additional axial T1-weighted
spin-echo images of the thoracic spine and a coronal STIR sequence
of the lumbar spine to include the pelvis.

FINDINGS:
The patient has had a recent orchiectomy (approximately five
weeks ago) and has also had radiation therapy to the pelvis.

Cervical Spine: Decreased signal intensity in marrow, consistent
with metastatic disease, is seen involving multiple levels,
predominantly in the odontoid, at C5 and C6 and T2 and T3.
Lamina and spinous processes also show some involvement, but
there is no expansion either in the vertebral bodies or other
elements of the cervical spine that narrows the canal or
compromises the cord.

Thoracic Spine: As in the cervical spine, scattered metastases
are evident with the most prominent involvement being at T4, T5,
T8 and T9 and T11. As in the cervica spine, there is also
involvement of posterior elements, but no expansion of marrow
space seen to compromise the canal or cord. However, there is
subtly increased signal intensity in and around the thecal sac,
seen on axial images, that is difficult to define as artifact or
possibly leptomeningeal metastases. A number of the axial images
show some motion degradation, but this questionable thickening o
meninges around the cord can be seen on virtually all axial images
on sheet 4/5. Again, there is no distortion or displacement of
the cord nor any alteration of the normal contours of the thecal
sac to clearly identify this as abnormal and it is not seen in the
cervical or lumbosacral region.

Lumbosacral Spine/Sacrum: Metastatic involvement in the
lumbosacral spine predominates at L2 and L3, but scattered foci
are also seen at L1 and L4. Fatty changes are seen in marrow of
L5 and within the sacrum, consistent with the patient having had
prior radiation.

(CONTINUED)

1001 Boylston Avenue   Seattle, Washington 98104   206/329-MRMR (6767)   FAX# 206/323-6989

FIRST HILL

DIAGNOSTIC
IMAGING
CENTER

R(, V
DOB: 09/23/20
SEX: M
6642

MR OF THE CERVICAL, THORACIC & LUMBAR SPINE: 11/21/91

(CONTINUED - PAGE 2)

A small focal (1 cm diameter) area of increased signal intensity
on coronal STIR images of the lumbar spine and sacrum, seen on
coronal STIR images C7 through C9 (2/5) may be a small area of
treated, now necrotic tumor, but that this is residual or
recurrent metastatic disease cannot be completely excluded.

The lumbosacral spinal canal is of normal caliber and no
findings are seen to suggest compromise of the thecal sac or
nerve roots.

IMPRESSION:
1.   Questionable meningeal thickening is seen in the thoracic
spine, but it is unclear whether this is real or might reflect
some scanning artifact. This was discussed with the referring
physician and the patient will be rescheduled for a limited
follow-up study without and with intravenous gadolinium to
answer this question.

2.   Cervical Spine: No cord- or canal-compromising lesions seen.

3.   Lumbosacral Spine: No canal-, cord-, or root-compromising
lesions identified.

4.   Diffuse bony metastatic disease is seen in the cervical,
thoracic, and lumbosacral spine. However, at no point is there
marrow expansion to compromise the spinal canal or neural
foramina. Fatty change is seen in the L5 vertebral body and the
sacrum consistent with radiation therapy. A 1 cm in diameter
focus of increased signal intensity in the mid-inferior right
ilium may reflect treated, now nonviable tumor, but that this is
due to persistent viable tumor or recurrent disease cannot be
completely excluded.

JWB/glh
Referring Physician:
MEHMET FER, M.D.

JAMES W. BORROW, M.D.

1001 Boylston Avenue   Seattle, Washington 98104   206/329-MRMR (6767)   FAX# 206/323-6989

FiRST HiLL

DIAGNOSTIC
IMAGING
CENTER

R   VI
DOB: 09/23/20
SEX: M
6642

MR THORACIC SPINE WITH GADOLINIUM: 11/23/91

70447008

CLINICAL HISTORY:

Patient with prostatic carcinima and known bony metastases.
Question of leptomeningeal metastases on recent noncontrast
magnetic resonance scan of the spine. Further evaluation with
intravenous contrast.

TECHNIQUE:

Sagittal and axial T1-weighted spin-echo sequences of the
thoracic spine before and after the intravenous administration of
13 ml of gadopentatate dimeglumine as contrast. Consent for the
use of intravenous contrast was signed before the study.

FINDINGS:

Axial T1-weighted spin-echo images done before the intravenous
administration of gadolinium are moderately motion-degraded.
However, sagittal pre and post and axial post-contrast scans are
almost completely motion-free.

Please see the earlier report (11/21/91) for details concerning
the extensive bony spinal metastases in this patient. As was
noted in the earlier report, however, there is no expansion of
marrow-based disease to compromise the thoracic spinal canal.

No findings are seen to suggest leptomeningeal or epidural
metastases on today's pre- and post-gadolinium-enhanced
sequences. The canal and cord are of normal caliber, and no
enhancing material is seen within the canal or the thecal sac,
nor is there any thickening of meninges to suggest the presence
of tumor.

IMPRESSION:

1. Extensive spinal bony metastases as previously described.   No
expansion of marrow disease to compromise canal, cord, or neural
foramina.

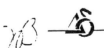

(CONTINUED)

1001 Boylston Avenue   Seattle, Washington 98104   206/329-MRMR (6767)   FAX# 206/323-6989

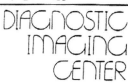

FIRST HILL
DIAGNOSTIC
IMAGING
CENTER

```
I       ,
DOB: 09/23/20
SEX: M
6642
```

MR THORACIC SPINE WITH GADOLINIUM: **11/23/91**

(CONTINUED - PAGE 2)

2. No signs of epidural or meningeal metastatic disease as seen
on pre- or post-gadolinium-enhanced sequences. I think that the
questionable abnormalities seen on the study from 11/21/91 were
artifacts induced by patient motion, with blurring and increased
signal intensity transmitted into the thecal space and canal to
mimic meningeal thickening and increased signal within the
epidural space.

JWB/mdb
Referring Physician:
MEHMET FER, M.D.

JAMES W. BORROW, M.D.

1001 Boylston Avenue   Seattle, Washington 98104   206/329-MRMR (6767)   FAX# 206/323-6989

Renal Cell Carcinoma

23. Patient RE
DOB: 7/27/24

Patient RE is a 68 year-old white male with a history of metastatic renal cell carcinoma. Patient RE had previously been in excellent health when in October of 1990 he was noted to have an abdominal mass on a routine physical examination. Patient RE was then referred for MRI and CT scan studies, which both revealed a 14 cm. tumor in the left kidney, with no evidence of metastases. Chest X-ray and bone scan were clear. Subsequently, on October 26, 1990, he went for exploratory laparotomy and left nephrectomy. The pathology report indicates renal cell carcinoma, with 1/1 adjacent nodes positive for invasive cancer.

On December 20, 1990, Patient RE began an experimental protocol with alpha-interferon administered at New York University Medical Center. The regimen ended in August of 1991, after eight months of treatment.

Thereafter, Patient RE did well until late November of 1991, when he noticed a lump behind his right ear that rapidly increased in size over a period of days. On December 5, 1991, fine needle aspiration revealed adenocarcinoma consistent with metastatic renal tubular adenocarcinoma. CT of the head on 12/9/91 documented a lytic lesion in the left parietal bone with an associated enhancing soft tissue mass and intracranial extension as well as extension into the subcutaneous tissue. CT of the abdomen and chest were negative, except for several questionable pulmonary nodules that were thought to represent vasculature. Bone scan was consistent with metastasis to the skull.

Patient RE then began a one-month course of radiation to the mass, totaling 4000 rads and completed on January 23, 1992. The tumor regressed only slightly during the therapy.

Patient RE learned of my work and realizing the severity of his situation, decided to pursue my protocol. I first saw him in my office on January 30, 1992 and at that time, he reported about a 20-pound weight loss over a period of six weeks. In addition, his orange-sized left parietal area tumor was immediately obvious. He was taking Allopurinol 300 mg QD.

Patient RE began his nutritional protocol in February of 1992. Within weeks, he noted an improvement in his energy and well being, as well as a 20-pound weight gain. In addition, within three months on his protocol, the previously noted large skull mass had completely resolved. Today, Patient RE remains completely compliant with his treatment, is in excellent health and disease-free. When last seen in June of 1993, he had no complaints.

Dr. Gonzalez presented these 25 cancer case studies to the NCI in 1993 and then updated the patient status information in 2001. Below are Dr. Gonzalez's personal notes with updated survival information:

Stage IV kidney cancer. Alive and well 9 years out.

Mr Kuvrn 14 5'3 /110 lbs

1.53 M²

WHITE PLAINS HOSPITAL MEDICAL CENTER
SURGICAL PATHOLOGY
SIGNED-OUT REPORT
SHALIT M.D.,SHIMON (177) —— 914-948 3128

PAGE 1
FOR: OCT 29, 1!

914 651 0600

α Dr Lipman
11/1/90

R. ,E: 8098287 (U:326908) 66 M ICUF06 ICU
======================

90-S07150R COLL: 10/26/90 3:00 PM RECV: 10/26/90 3:15 PM

PHYSICIAN(S): SHALIT M.D.,SHIMON (177)
COMMENT: A. LT RIB
         B. LT KIDNEY
         PATHOLOGIST DR. SABBIA
CLINICAL HISTORY: LT ABDOMINAL MASS
SURGICAL PROCEDURE(S): NEPHRECTOMY
TISSUE(S): LEFT KIDNEY
PROCEDURE(S): S TECHNICAL AND CLERICAL ASST., SURGICAL BLOCKS\9,
S HPS ROUTINE STAIN\9, EXTENSIVE COMPL. SPEC., DR. SABBIA, 189.0

GROSS DESCRIPTION: RFS:VM 10/29/

The specimen is received in two parts. The first consists of the
left 8th rib which measures 13 cm. in length and up to 1.5 cm. in
width. There is no gross change of significant note.

The main specimen consists of the left kidney measuring 23 x 14 x
15 cm. and weighing 2046 grams. The external surface is partially
covered by lobules of fat but is otherwise smooth, and dark
reddish-tan in color. No obvious tumor is visualized from the
surface. A small inferior pole of grossly unremarkable kidney is
seen which measures 4.5 cm x 4 cm. in its greatest dimension. The
fatty tissue is dissected away exposing the rim of a portion of
adrenal gland which is sectioned and submitted. This is otherwise
unremarkable. The area of the pelvis and initial portion of the
ureter measuring 3.5 cm. is identified with some surrounding
vessels. Sections are submitted labeled A and B. The portion of
adrenal gland is submitted labeled C. The tissue adjacent to this
is submitted labeled D. Upon opening and exposing the pelvic area
and vessels there is no gross evidence of any extension of tumor
into these structures. The specimen is then fully opened and a
gigantic necrotic, yellowish-tan tumor mass is exposed which
occupies the bulk of the kidney leaving a 6 cm. segment of
uninvolved parenchyma. It is from this latter area that the
intact and grossly uninvolved pelvis and ureter can be seen. The
tumor which reaches up to the renal capsule does not appear to
penetrate it in any area. Sections from the renal tumor are
submitted labeled E and section from the uninvolved parenchyma
labeled F. Sections from the surface of the kidney are submitted
labeled G.

```
  / 29, 1990         WHITE PLAINS HOSPITAL MEDICAL CENTER          PAGE 2
  :22 PM                      SURGICAL PATHOLOGY             FOR: OCT 29, 19
                             SIGNED-OUT REPORT
                        SHALIT M.D.,SHIMON (177)
```

RU: ,E.   6098287 (U:326908)   66 M ICUF06 ICU
========================

MICRO EXAMINATION: RFS:VM 10/29/9

Sections A and B reveal portions of ureter and sections through
numerous vessels representing the major vascular structures at the
hilum of the kidney. These are all free of tumor.

Sections C reveal a portion of uninvolved adrenal gland.

Sections D reveal a lymph node with microscopic deposits of tumor.

Sections E reveal various areas through primarily necrotic renal
tissue however foci of well-preserved cellularity is seen and here
one can identify a tubular-type pattern with malignant epithelial
cells.

Sections F reveal uninvolved portions of kidney.

Section G reveals additional fragments of fibromuscular stroma and
vessels negative for tumor.

                       ** FINAL DIAGNOSES **
                       ========================

MICROSCOPIC DIAGNOSIS:
RENAL CELL CARCINOMA OF LEFT KIDNEY.
RENAL VESSELS, NEGATIVE FOR MALIGNANCY.
PORTION OF ADRENAL GLAND.
ONE REGIONAL LYMPH NODE POSITIVE FOR MALIGNANCY.
PORTION OF LEFT RIB.
88309
189.0
<RFS:VM 10/29/90>

=> SIGNED OUT BY: RICHARD F. SABBIA M.D. --------------------- 10/29/90
```
```

NEW YORK UNIVERSITY MEDICAL CENTER

Tisch Hospital
560 First Avenue

Department of Pathology
New York, NY '10016

(212) 263-5470

SURGICAL PATHOLOGY CONSULTATION

ASPIRATION BIOPSY

PATIENT: R   ,E

ADDRESS:

ACCESSION #:   **FNA91-392**

MED REC #: UNKNOWN
BIRTHDATE: 07/27/24 (Age: 67)
SEX: M
PHYSICIAN: Ronald Blum, M.D.

SERVICE: Medicine
PATIENT TYPE: Outpatient Chargeable
DATE ACCESSIONED: 12/05/91

HISTORY:
Radiotherapy: N   Chemotherapy: N Prior Operations: Left nephrectomy,
2 hernia repairs Surgical No: N Infections: N Prior Cytology: N
Mammograms: N

Comments: 1 -------- Lymph node - perirenal

SOURCE(S) OF SPECIMEN:
Scalp mass

****
FINAL DIAGNOSIS:

SKIN, SCALP, LEFT OCCIPITAL AREA: ASPIRATION
  - ADENOCARCINOMA, CONSISTENT WITH METASTATIC RENAL TUBULAR
ADENOCARCINOMA.

                              Jerry Waisman, M.D.

              ** Report Electronically Signed Out **
****
DESCRIPTION OF PROCEDURE AND MICROSCOPIC FINDINGS:
Dr. Waisman explained the procedure to Mr. R   and with his permission
twice aspirated a 1 cm soft ill-defined left suboccipital nodule using 27
gauge needles. The area felt soft during aspiration. There was no
unusual pain. The aspirates were bloody. Four smears were prepared for
Diff-quik and H&E stains. The smears showed blood and many large atypical
epithelial cells, singly and in clusters. Papillary structures were
evident. The atypical cells had vacuolated cytoplasm and prominent
nucleoli. There was necrotic debris.

                              Jerry Waisman, M.D.

OF SLIDES: 4

continued...   REPORTED DATE: 12/11/91

(212) 263-7216

FACULTY PRACTICE RADIOLOGY
530 FIRST AVENUE
NEW YORK, NEW YORK 10016

December 9, 1991

Ronald Blum, M.D.
530 First Avenue
Suite 4J
New York, NY 10016

                    Re: E   R

Dear Doctor Blum:

The following is a radiologic consultation on your patient:

COMPUTED TOMOGRAPHY OF THE BRAIN

Axial CT images of the brain were obtained from base to
vertex following the intravenous administration of contrast
material.

There is a lytic lesion within the left parietal bone with
an associated enhancing soft tissue mass, consistent with
a metastasis. There is intracranial extension of the enhancing soft tissue, as well as extension into the subcutaneous tissue of the left parietal scalp.

There is a rounded collection of material of identical
attenuation to the cerebrospinal fluid within the posterior
portion of the posterior fossa, located in the midline and
to the left, most consistent with an arachnoid cyst. This
arachnoid cysts measures approximately 2.8cm in greatest
diameter.

There is no evidence of intracranial hemorrhage, hydrocephalus, or midline shift.

(cont'd. on pg. #2)

-1-

(212) 263-7216

FACULTY PRACTICE RADIOLOGY
530 FIRST AVENUE
NEW YORK, NEW YORK 10016

December 9, 1991

Doctor Ronald Blum   Re: E   R

(cont'd. from pg. #1)

IMPRESSION.

1. Lytic lesion within the left parietal bone with an asso-
    ciated enhancing soft tissue mass, consistent with a
    metastasis. There is intracranial extension of the
    enhancing soft tissue mass.

2. Posterior fossa arachnoid cyst.

Thank you for referring this patient for consultation.

                Sincerely yours,

                MICHEAL HARNED, M.D.
                JEFFREY WEINREB, M.D.

MH:JW:mlm
12/11/91

-2-

Sarcoma

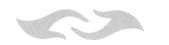

24. Patient CS
DOB: 5/27/64

Patient CS is a 29 year-old white female with a long history of alveolar soft cell sarcoma, initially diagnosed in May 1977 when she developed a left thigh tumor. The lesion was resected, and after a negative metastatic workup, she received 6000 rads to the tumor bed, followed by a one-year course of chemotherapy with Vincristine, Cytoxan and actinomycin D. She subsequently did well until 1987, when she developed pain under her left scapula. Her doctors initially thought the symptoms insignificant, but when Patient CS developed left neck swelling she underwent an evaluation at Kaiser Permanente Hospital in April 1988. She was found to have a soft tissue mass in the inferior aspect of the scapula with muscle invasion, and chest X-ray revealed four pulmonary nodules consistent with metastatic disease.

A biopsy of the scapular lesion on April 28, 1988 demonstrated recurrent alveolar cell sarcoma. At that time, Patient CS began chemotherapy with adriamycin and DTIC, but when repeat chest X-ray showed no improvement after three cycles, the treatment was discontinued. The sarcoma group at Stanford told her and her family that she suffered a very aggressive, treatment resistant cancer, and she most likely had no more than 3–6 months to live.

Patient CS learned of my work and was initially seen in my office on October 3, 1988. She denied any symptoms at that time, and her exam was notable for a 6 cm. hard, fixed tumor in the left scapular area.

Upon returning to California, Patient CS began her nutritional protocol. A chest X-ray from October 28, 1988, three weeks after Patient CS began her program, describes "Three well defined lung masses. Largest in lingula, measuring 2.4 by 2.2 cm. Two smaller well circumscribed masses in the right lower lobe seen best on the lateral view. Large lytic focus along inferior margin of left scapula near tip, about 3 cm. in length."

For at least the first six months on the protocol, Patient CS was by her and her family's description, very compliant with her nutritional protocol, and sequential X-rays of her lungs documented improvement in her pulmonary nodules after an initial period of stabilization. An X-ray from November 30, 1988 described "Three nodules, unchanged since prior film: lytic lesion scapula unchanged since prior film." A chest X-ray on March 2, 1989 again showed stabilization, with little change, reported as:

"Left lung nodule measuring 2.3 by 2.8 cm.: two smaller right pulmonary masses seen best on lateral and not significantly changed. Left scapular lesion unchanged."

Then, three months later, on June 6, 1989, an X-ray showed resolution of one tumor and reduction in the other two, as documented in the official report:

"Two nodules as previously described. Left midlung nodule measures 2.5 by 2.0 cm., smaller than when compared to previous studies. Nodular density in the right lower lung field 1.9 by 1.5 cm. and slightly smaller if anything. Left scapula unchanged."

At that time, Patient CS felt so well her parents allowed her to go to England for a two-month vacation. Unfortunately, during this time she went off her diet and protocol completely. Not surprisingly, after Patient CS returned to California, a chest X-ray dated September 19, 1989 showed enlargement of the right pulmonary nodule.

When Patient CS returned to my office on October 5, 1989, I talked to her about the need for compliance. Thereafter, for a period of about six months, she was very dedicated to her protocol, but during the summer of 1990, she again became careless. Without my knowledge, in July of 1990 Patient CS entered American International Hospital in Zion, Illinois for chemotherapy. Subsequently, Patient CS said she deceived herself into looking for a simple answer to her disease. At American International, she received a single course of ifosphamide, which made her very ill but did nothing for her tumors. She signed herself out, and went back on her nutritional protocol.

Since that time, her course has been erratic, characterized by periods of full compliance followed by periods of total non-compliance. During the latter part of 1992, she was mostly off her protocol, and her scapular tumor increased in size. In February 1993, after an episode of hemoptysis, Patient CS was told by her local physicians that she was "dying," and needed immediate radiation therapy. After a single dose, she called me from her hospital bed, and I again lectured her about the need to follow her program as prescribed. Patient CS declined further radiation, signed herself out and restarted her nutritional protocol. She quickly stabilized, and did well enough to come to my office in June of 1993 for a re-evaluation. At that time, she said her scapula lesion was shrinking and her breathing had become "normal." She seems to be fully compliant and doing better, nearly five years after beginning her nutritional therapy.

Patient CS is an interesting patient for a number of reasons. She is her own control, doing well when she follows her program, suffering disease progression when she is non-compliant. In her defense, she has been fighting cancer for 16 years, and gets "tired of it all," as she says. At times, she just wants to lead a normal life, free even of the restraints of my program. But, despite her rocky course, she is still alive, currently stable despite dire warnings from many physicians, and has long ago outlived the prognosis given her at Stanford.

Dr. Gonzalez presented these 25 cancer case studies to the NCI in 1993 and then updated the patient status information in 2001. Below are Dr. Gonzalez's personal notes with updated survival information:

Metastatic Stage IV sarcoma. Had regression of disease but quit after 5 years and eventually died.

ELEVEN-ELEVEN SONOMA AVENUE X-RAY

1111 SONOMA AVENUE • SUITE 112 • SANTA ROSA, CA 95405 • (707) 526-2935

Radiologists: Robert L. Scheibel, M.D.; Gordon Witwer, M.D.; Shirley E. Beshany, M.D.; Douglas A. Munro, M.D.

REPORT OF EXAMINATION

NAME: C   , S

Address:

Phone:

Date: 10-28-88
X-RAY NO.:   18428
D.O.B.   5-27-64
Dr.   H. Richardson

Examination of:

CHEST, PA AND LATERAL:

Clinical History:

Illegible.

Two views obtained of the chest compared with the previous examination dated 9-21-88.

There are three well defined lung masses seen in the lung. The largest is in the lingula and measures 2.4 x 2.2 cm. There are two smaller well circumscribed masses identified in the right lower lobe seen best on the lateral examination, one being just below the hilum and the other being in the costophrenic angle posteriorly. These are unchanged in size and appearance since the last examination and likely represents metastasis. The remainder of the lung parenchyma, pulmonary vascularity and cardiomediastinal silhouette appears normal. There is again noted the large lytic focus seen along the inferior margin of the left scapula near the tip. This measures approximately 3 cm in length and is likely unchanged since the previous examination. Small calcific/ossific densities are seen within the adjoining soft tissues. It is unclear if this represents displaced bone trabecula or if there is distrophic calcification secondary to therapy. No other bony lesions are identified.

IMPRESSION: No significant change with bilateral lung
               metastases.

               Probably no change in left scapular metastasis.

Thank you for this referral.

DOUGLAS MUNRO, M.D.
Radiologist

DM:plc
D&T: 10-31-88

ELEVEN-ELEVEN SONOMA AVENUE X-RAY

1111 SONOMA AVENUE • SUITE 112 • SANTA ROSA, CA 95405 • (707) 526-2935

Radiologists: Robert L. Scheibel, M.D.; Gordon Witwer, M.D.; Shirley E. Beshany, M.D.; Douglas A. Munro, M.D.

REPORT OF EXAMINATION

NAME: C   S

Address:

Phone:

Date: 11-30-88

X-RAY NO.   18428

D.O.B.   5-27-64

Dr.   H. Richardson

Examination of: **CHEST, PA AND LATERAL:**

Clinical History: Sarcoma.

PA and lateral views of the chest demonstrate a lesion at the tip of the left scapula. Compared to the previous film of 10-28-88, there has been no change. There is a nodular density seen in the left midlung field. There are two nodular densities seen in the right lower lung fields. These are unchanged when compared to the previous exam.

The remainder of the lung fields are clear of acute infiltration, consolidation or effusion. The cardiac and mediastinal silhouettes appear normal. Compared to the previous film, there has been no change.

IMPRESSION: No significant change.

Thank you for this referral.

SHIRLEY BESHANY, M.D.
Radiologist

SB:plc
D: 11-30-88
T: 12-1-88

ELEVEN-ELEVEN SONOMA AVENUE X-RAY

1111 SONOMA AVENUE • SUITE 112 • SANTA ROSA, CA 95405 • (707) 526-2935

Radiologists: Robert L. Scheibel, M.D.; Gordon Witwer, M.D.; Shirley E. Beshany, M.D.; Douglas A. Munro, M.D.

REPORT OF EXAMINATION

NAME:
      C.   S

Address:

Phone:

Date: 3-2-89
X-RAY NO.
D.O.B.   18428
        5-27-64
Dr.   H. Richardson

Examination of:

      CHEST AND LEFT SCAPULA.

Clinical History:

      Sarcoma.

Erect PA and lateral views of the chest show the cardiac, mediastinal
and hilar contours to be normal. The lungs are normally inflated.
Again noted are three pulmonary nodules, the largest is in the left
midlung field and has increased slightly in size from previous
examinations, now measuring 23 x 28 mm in size. Two smaller soft tissue
nodules are present in the right lower lobe medially, which are not
significantly changed from prior examinations. No new pulmonary nodules
or infiltrates are demonstrated, no pleural fluid is present.

Both the chest radiograph and coned down views of the scapula
demonstrate an area of irregular bony destruction combined with areas
of new bone formation at the tip of the scapula. This is unchanged from
prior examinations and probably indicates a bony metastatic deposit. No
new lesions are demonstrated.

CONCLUSION: Chest x-ray again demonstrates bilateral pulmonary
                nodules as described above with very slight interval
                enlargement of the left pulmonary nodule.

                The left scapular lesion is unchanged and no new bony
                lesions are demonstrated.

Thank you for this referral.

                          GORDON WITWER, M.D.
                          Radiologist

GW:plc
D: 3-3-89
T: 3-6-89

0

ELEVEN-ELEVEN SONOMA AVENUE X-RAY

1111 SONOMA AVENUE • SUITE 112 • SANTA ROSA, CA 95405 • (707) 526-2935

Radiologists: Robert L. Scheibel, M.D.; Gordon Witwer, M.D.; Shirley E. Beshany, M.D.; Douglas A. Munro, M.D.

REPORT OF EXAMINATION

NAME: C.   S.

Address:

Phone:

Date: 6-6-89
X-RAY NO. 18428
D.O.B.   5-27-64
Dr.   H. Richardson

Examination of: **CHEST, PA AND LATERAL:**

Clinical History: Sarcoma with metastases.

Compare to multiple previous films dating back through 10-28-88 and a chest x-ray done at Kaiser Clinics in Santa Rosa dated 9-21-88.

The two previously described nodular densities are again identified. The larger of the two densities located in the left midlung field projecting over the tip of the fourth rib. This nodular density measures 25 x 20 mm and is smaller than when compared to previous multiple studies. The nodular density in the right lower lung field projecting over the posterior aspect of the eleventh rib measures 19 x 15 mm and is also stable and if anything, slightly smaller. There are no new nodular densities noted. The other incidental changes are again identified with the cardiomediastinal structures, pleural surfaces being intact and normal. The bony changes over the tip of the left scapula with sclerosis and relative healing is again noted and unchanged.

CONCLUSION: Stable pulmonary nodule slightly different in size, if anything smaller. No evidence for new nodules and no evidence for enlargement of the existing nodules.

Stable bony focus of metastases involving the inferior angle of the left scapula. This lesion shows healing and certainly no progression.

Summary: Radiographically the patient is stable and in fact slightly improving.

Thank you for this referral.

Thanks.

ROBERT SCHEIBEL, M.D.
Radiologist

RS:plc
D&T: 6-7-89

ELEVEN-ELEVEN SONOMA AVENUE X-RAY

1111 SONOMA AVENUE • SUITE 112 • SANTA ROSA, CA 95405 • (707) 526-2935

Radiologists: Robert L. Scheibel, M.D.; Gordon Witwer, M.D.; Shirley E. Beshany, M.D.; Douglas A. Munro, M.D.

REPORT OF EXAMINATION

NAME: C.   S   Date: 9-19-89

                                                                             X-RAY NO.   18428

Address: D.O.B.   5-27-64

Phone: Dr.   H. Richardson

Examination of: **CHEST, PA AND LATERAL:**

Clinical History: 25 year old woman who recently had a soft tissue
                       sarcoma removed from the tip of the left scapula.
                       Patient has been on various therapy including
                       secondary types of therapy.

Compare to 6-6-89.

There is a normal inspiratory effort. The diaphragms project
down to the tenth posterior rib. The trachea and mediastinal
structures are in midline position with symmetrical aeration.
The two previously described nodular densities demonstrated
in the film of 6-6-89 are again identified. Allowing for
slight differences in technique, the nodular density in the
left midlung field projecting over the anterior arc of the
fourth left rib is not significantly changed in size and
configuration. The nodular density projecting in the right
lower lobe and over the posterior arc of the eleventh rib
is, if anything, very slightly larger or certainly the same
size. No new nodular densities are identified. The irregularity of the tip of the left scapula is again identified.
This is not changed. However, the left breast shadow appears
to be slightly larger than the right. I am not certain why
this is. The bony thorax is intact. The heart, aorta and
pulmonary vessels are normal.

CONCLUSION: Two large pulmonary nodules as described above.
               Overall there has been no significant or dramatic
               change in the size or configuration of the nodules
               when compared to the film of 6-6-89. However,
               when compared to the film of 10-28-88 there
has been an increase in particular in the size of the right
lower lobe nodule.

Thank you for this referral.

                                    ROBERT SCHEIBEL, M.D.
                                    Radiologist

RS:plc
D&T: 9-19-89

KAISER FOUNDATION HOSPITALS

OPERATION RECORD

PATIENT		MEDICAL RECORD NUMBER
C S		
BIRTHDATE	ROOM 522	DATE 9-28-77

PRE-OPERATIVE DIAGNOSIS: LEFT ANTEROLATERAL THIGH MASS

POST-OPERATIVE DIAGNOSIS: LEFT ANTEROLATERAL THIGH MASS

OPERATION: EXCISION OF LEFT ANTEROLATERAL THIGH MASS

FINDINGS: Encapsulated 3 x 4 cm. firm red-brown tissue.

PROCEDURE: Under general anesthesia the patient was prepped and draped in a normal sterile fashion. Longitudinal incision was made in the left anterolateral thigh approximately 5 cms. long 10 cms. above the left patella, 4 cms. to the left of midline. The excision was carried down thru the fascia lata to the vastus lateralis muscle. Hemostasis was achieved with the Bovie. A firm, approximately 3 x 4 cm. encapsulated mass was then palpated and neatly excised with the use of the Bovie cutting edge. Tissue was forwarded to pathology for identification. The muscle bed space was then closed with 3-0 plain and the fascia lata closed with 3-0 Dexon, subcutaneous tissue closed with 3-0 plain and subcuticular sutures of 4-0 Dexon were placed in a symmetric fashion. The skin was closed with running 4-0 nylon sutures. Estimated blood loss 15 ccs.

PROCEDURE: Complications: none. Fluid: D-5 acetated Ringer's. Patient tolerated the procedure well and was returned to the PAR in stable condition.

Surgeons: Bruce May, M.D., Resident

Ian Leverton, M.D., Resident

Richard Geist, M.D.

BM:mb
Dict. 9-28-77
Trans. 9-28-77

SURGEON

90511 (REV 2-71)

240

| ☐ GROSS PHOTOS ☐ MIRCO PHOTOS | **PATHOLOGY CONSULTATION REPORT** KAISER-PERMANENTE MEDICAL CENTER LABORATORY 77 | | PATHOLOGY ACCESSION NO. (57-64) **RS77-4447** |

DR.	FACILITY/LOC.	☐OUTPAT.	DATE 9-28-77	LAST NAME	FIRST	INITIAL
TISSUE	TISSUE SITE	☐INPAT.	ROOM NO. 512	BIRTHDATE ... C ...		
CLINICAL DATA (INCLUDING PREVIOUS PATH NOS., CLINICAL DX, LMP)				MEDICAL ID CARD NUMBER (65-72) 05 66 ... 3 1371960		
				SEX (73) ☐M ☐F	COVERAGE AGE (73-75) 83 463 1382550	0
		PAP TAKEN WITH THIS BIOPSY? ☐ YES		O/P REVENUE SLIP NO.	AMOUNT $	☐ CASH ☐ CHARGE RECPT.

SPACE BELOW RESERVED FOR PATHOLOGIST

GROSS; Received in formalin labeled "mass of right thigh" is a brown red rounded soft fragment of tissue weighing 9 gms. and measuring 4 cm. x 3 cm. Within this mass of brown tissue is a rounded tan brown well-demarcated nodule measuring 2 cm. x 2 cm. x 2.5 cm. Rep. sections as A, B, and C.

MICRO: Micro. sections show tumor in skeletal muscle which is forming alveoli and contains very large cells with bizarre nuclei and eosinophilic cytoplasm. Delicate fibrous septae separate the alveoli with capillaries running through it. The tumor presses into surrounding skeletal muscle and is also seen within blood vessels.

This tumor has been known by many names and its cell of origin is disputed. These tumors have been thought to arise from vascular glomera of paraganglia (malignant nonchromaffin paraganglioma); skeletal muscle (rhabdomyosarcoma or polymorphous sarcoma); from myoblasts (malignant granular cell

-2-   RS77-4447

myoblastoma); or of undetermined origin (alveolar soft part and sarcoma - a descriptive term). They are relatively uncommon/are prone to occur in adolescents and young adults with females being affected more than males. They usually occur in an extremity, often the lower extremities, although they can occur in the abdominal wall, perianal region, tongue, floor of mouth, and orbit. It may recur locally following simple excision; radical excision or amputation is the usual method of treatment. Pulmonary cerebral and skeletal metastases occur in more than 50% of cases.

MICRO. DIAG: X ALVEOLAR SOFT PART SARCOMA (EXCISION FROM LEFT THIGH).

K.A. GRICE, M.D. (C)

97682 (REV. 8-76)   DOCTOR'S COPY

☐ GROSS PHOTOS
☐ MICRO PHOTOS
Hoffman

PATHOLOGY CONSULTATION REPORT

KAISER-PERMANENTE MEDICAL CENTER LABORATORY

PATHOLOGY ACCESSION NO. (57-64)

RS88-4759

DR. _Hoffman_   FACILITY/LOCI _OFFEN_   ☐ OUTPAT.   DATE 4/26/88   ☐ INPAT.

TISSUE   TISSUE SITE _mass left back_   ROOM NO. 419B

CLINIC   DX

PAP TAKEN WITH THIS BIOPSY?   ☐ YES

O/P REVENUE SLIP NO.   AMOUNT $ ☐ CASH ☐ CHARGE RECPT.

3 1371960

SPACE BELOW RESERVED FOR PATHOLOGIST

4/26/88 P/c
GROSS:

2 x 1.5 x 1 cm red brown soft tissue containing a gray-pink fleshy tumor mass. Three slides of imprints are saved for possible Wright Giemsa stain. All A and B.

MICRO DESCRIPTION: Sections of soft tissue mass from left back show histologic pattern the same as seen in the previous lesion RS77-4447 and represents an alveolar soft parts sarcoma. This present lesion has a lobulated pattern and it interdigitates between fascia and skeletal muscle. There are foci of metaplastic bone formation present. The initial report in 1977 states that the lesion was located in the thigh, thus this must represent a metastases, although I have no idea if it is in the locale of her previous lesion. In any event, the mass represents an alveolar soft part sarcoma and extends to all margins of the biopsy.

Page 2   RS88-4759

MICRO DIAGNOSIS: ALVEOLAR SOFT PART SARCOMA, MASS, LEFT BACK.

T 4/28/88 r 4759   B.J. SCHREINER, M.D.
RVS 88305

DATE COMPLETED

DATE RECEIVED

242

SEX	PATIENT NAME			M.R. NUMBER	AGE		IMPRINT AREA

Patient Name: C____ S____ M
M.R. NUMBER: 371960 AGE: 23
BIRTHDATE: 05/27/64

COV: S3 GROUP: 00463 ACCOUNT: 1382550

HOME ADDRESS: CA 95401
SOURCE OF PAYMENT: 01 SMOKER: NO M.S.: S RACE: 5 RELIGION: NON

VALUABLES: NO MEDS: NO

SUBSCRIBER'S NAME: C____ W____ O
SUBSCRIBER'S EMPLOYER: MARIN CO EMP

LAST KFH ADMISSION: SRF ON 08/22/86
ADMITTING PHYSICIAN: P G HOFFMAN M.D.
ATTENDING PHYSICIAN: P G HOFFMAN M.D.

OTHER INSURANCE: MEDICARE

SRF 008833

ADMISSION
TIME: 08:07 DATE ADMITTED: 04/26/88 JULIAN DAY: 17 TYPE ADM: C

DISCHARGE
TIME: 1210 DATE DISCHARGED: 4-28-88 JULIAN DAY: 119 TOTAL HOSP DAYS: 2

UNIT: 4EAS ROOM NO: A19 BED: B PROF. SERV.: SURG

USUAL PHYSICIAN: HOFFMAN S HOFFMAN M.D.
OUTPATIENT CARE FACILITY: SRO

EMERGENCY CONTACTS / RELATION NAME: P BILL AND LEE C
707-579-8344
ADMITTING CLERK: J MONTOOTH

ADMITTING DIAGNOSIS: SARCOMA L. BACK
SURGERY: INCISIONAL BX OF TUMOR LEFT BACK ON 04/26 AT 09:00

WORK RELATED: NO

PRINCIPAL DIAGNOSIS

MASS, LEFT BACK
Pathology report: Alveolar soft part sarcoma, mass, left back.

SECONDARY DIAGNOSIS OR COMPLICATIONS

INTRAOPERATIVE HEMORRHAGE

PRINCIPAL PROCEDURE

INCISIONAL BIOPSY, LEFT BACK TUMOR

TRANSFUSION

CONSULTANTS

RESULTS			AUTOPSY		CORONER CASE	
☐ DISCHARGED	☐ DISCHARGED AGAINST MEDICAL ADVICE	☐ EXPIRED	☐ YES	☐ NO	☐ YES	☐ NO

COMPLETED BY _____ M.D.   ATTENDING PHYSICIAN _____

Thyroid Cancer

25. Patient SM
DOB: 10/18/49

Patient SM is a 43 year-old white female harpist from Ohio with a history of both Hodgkin's disease and thyroid carcinoma. In May of 1964, when Patient SM was 14 years old, a biopsy of a persistently swollen left cervical lymph node revealed Hodgkin's lymphoma. In early July 1964, Patient SW was referred to M.D. Anderson Hospital in Houston, where physicians confirmed the diagnosis of Hodgkin's. In addition, chest Xrays demonstrated enlarged lymph nodes in the area of the left mediastinum and in the center of the left lung.

Patient SM then completed a fourweek course of cobalt radiation totaling 4000 rads to the neck and 4000 to the chest. At the conclusion of the treatment in midAugust, 1964, she was thought to be in remission.

Thereafter, Patient SM did well until early November of 1967, when she developed large masses in the left axilla and right clavicular region. After biopsy studies documented recurrent Hodgkin's disease, Patient SM received, at M.D. Anderson, an additional 4200 rads of cobalt radiation to the neck and chest. Once again, the disease regressed.

After this second episode, Patient SM appeared to be cancerfree until December of 1971 when, while attending college, she noted swelling along the length of her right arm. She also experienced shortness of breath, and left rib pain.

Patient SM returned to the outpatient clinic at M.D. Anderson, where, on physical exam, a large, 5 cm. mass in the left axilla was clearly evident. A chest Xray revealed thickening in the left pleura, as well as suspicious lesions in the seventh, eighth and ninth ribs.

Patient SM was readmitted to M.D. Anderson on January 18, 1972, for biopsy of the axillary mass, the pleura, and the left eighth rib. All tissue specimens were positive for Hodgkin's, nodular sclerosing type, confirming widespread, stage IV disease. The attending physicians recommended a sixmonth, sixcycle regimen of MOPP chemotherapy, which Patient SM began while still hospitalized. Initially, she tolerated the first cycle of drugs without serious side effects, but after returning home on January 29, she suffered nausea, frequent vomiting, and anorexia. Over a period of two weeks, she lost a total of 16 pounds.

Reluctantly, Patient SM returned to M.D. Anderson on February 20, 1972, for her second round of chemotherapy. She again became severely ill after the first infusion of medication and refused to proceed with treatment. At that time, she was not believed to be in remission.

Patient SM returned home, and resumed her college studies. At school, a friend who knew about Dr. Kelley gave her a copy of One Answer to Cancer. After reading the book, Patient SM set up and kept an appointment with Dr. Kelley, despite objections from her parents who believed Dr. Kelley to be a fraud.

Patient SM began the Kelley program in the spring of 1972, when she was not yet fully recovered from the effects of her chemotherapy. Over a period of many months, she regained her lost weight, and the chronic fatigue which had plagued her improved.

Patient SM continued the full Kelley regimen for two years, and then gradually adopted a maintenance protocol until discontinuing all nutritional treatment in the early 1980's. She remained in excellent health and cancer free until mid1986, when she developed a thyroid mass. Since the Kelley program was not at the time available, on August 20, 1986 Patient SM underwent partial resection of the thyroid. The pathology report described follicular carcinoma with evidence of vascular and carotid invasion, with multiple satellite lesions all over the submitted tissue.

Over the following two years, the tumor gradually regrew and Patient SM's physicians urged further surgery, to be followed by radiation and perhaps chemotherapy. But at that time, Patient SM had learned of my work and refused all further standard treatment.

Patient SM was first seen in my office on January 16, 1988 and at that time, she felt well. Her examination was notable for a 3 cm. hard non-tender right thyroid mass and right upper extremity lymphedema which has been present since lymphadenectomy done in the 1960's.

Upon returning to Ohio, Patient SM restarted her nutritional regimen that she has followed with great compliance. And over the years, her thyroid tumor has gradually resolved. When seen in my office on January 9, 1990, after she had been on her protocol two years, the thyroid mass had nearly completely regressed. A year later, on January 2, 1991, the mass was no longer palpable. When last seen in May of 1993, Patient SM was well, active, apparently disease free and an enthusiastic supporter of this protocol.

Dr. Gonzalez presented these 25 cancer case studies to the NCI in 1993 and then updated the patient status information in 2001. Below are Dr. Gonzalez's personal notes with updated survival information:

Thyroid cancer. An old Dr. Kelley patient who he cured of Hodgkin's disease. Alive and well 13 years since seeing me.

14x17_____ 7x17_____		ROUTINE REPORT	
14x14_____ 10x12_____			
11x14_____ 8x10_____	PLEASE USE PRESSURE WHEN WRITING	WET READING	
TECH_____		(CHECK ONE)	

FILM ORDERS (FOR USE OF RADIOLOGIST ONLY)

	CODING		
	1.	S˙ MISS M.	53343
	2.		
CHEST, PA AND LATERAL	3.	7-6-64	
	4.		
	5.	TO: MEDICAL RECORD	

PART TO BE EXAMINED:_____ CHEST, PA AND LATERAL

CLINICAL COMMENTS AND DIAGNOSIS:___ 6 mos. history of nuchal node enlargement, ciopsied in Amarillo
on June 23rd; diagnosed Hodgkin's Granuloma

_____ REQUESTING M. D.__ L. Moller

STRETCHER ☐   (CHECK ONE)
WHEEL CHAIR ☐   AMBULATORY ☐   HEIGHT_____WEIGHT_____AGE_____RACE_____SEX_____

ROENTGENOLOGICAL REPORT

FINDINGS:

CHEST: Examination of the chest by PA and lateral projections reveal
widening of the superior mediastinum on the left side measuring approximately 4.5 cm.
width from the mid line ~~at the~~ at the level of the posterior segment of the 6th rib on
projections. On the lateral projection, the mass appears to be located in the anterio
mediastinum. There is left hilar lymphadenopathy. The right hilar shadow appears nor
No evidence of active pneumonic process or neoplastic lesion is seen in either lung.fi
The heart is not enlarged. No pleural reaction is seen.

CONCLUSIONS: Left anterior mediastinal mass and left hilar lymphadenopathy
consistent with clinically known Hodgkin's disease.

DATE____7-6-64____   B. S. Jing/jp   M. D
                                                            RADIOLOGIST

THE UNIVERSITY OF TEXAS   DIAGNOSTIC ROENTGENOLOGY   6
M. D. ANDERSON HOSPITAL

THE UNIVERSITY OF TEXAS
M. D. ANDERSON HOSPITAL & TUMOR INSTITUTE
DEPARTMENT OF PATHOLOGY
Surgical Report

53343

Name: S   , M   Room: E 301 A   S-   72-0411

Unit No.:   Age: 23   Sex: Female   Race: White
Physician: Dr. Mountain   Service: Chest   Date: 1-19-72

Clinical Diagnosis:

Diagnosis and report
by: B. Mackay, M.D.

DIAGNOSIS:
(A) Pleural biopsy:
        Hodgkin's disease with nodular sclerosis
(B) Portion of 8th rib:
        Submitted for decalcification
(C) Node left axilla:
        Hodgkin's disease with nodular sclerosis

533-8891
535-8891

BM:kk:pb
S+2
1-21-72
1-21-72

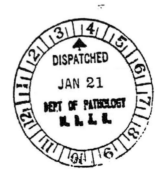

GRANDVIEW HOSPITAL - DEPARTMENT OF PATHOLOGY
405 GRAND AVENUE
DAYTON, OHIO 45405

Frank Brecher, D.O.-Chairman   Hosp. No. _____
Bernard Fox, D.O.-Associate
Patrocino Cruz, M.D.-Associate   Room No. _____

NAME   M   AGE 36   SEX F   SURG ____   ____

TISSUE TO BE EXAMINED: Thyroid Tissue; Portion of Anterior Jugular Vein

____palazs   ____   Forsh
       Surgeon   Referring Physician

BIOPSY NO.   S86-3785   8-20-   1986

GROSS EXAMINATION:

Submitted fresh for frozen section is a 5 x 3.5 x 1.5 cm., .15 gms. multilobular
thyroid tissue. Serial sections reveal a 1.5 cm. hemorrhagic nodule and a 1 cm. a
smooth nodule. Two sections submitted for frozen.

                         B. Kitchener, M.D.

In formalin is a 2 cm long tubular structure with a scant amount of fibrofatty
tissue. Sectioning shows a lumen partially filled with blood clot. A
representative section is submitted.

                         Patrocino Cruz, M.D.

MICROSCOPIC EXAMINATION:

Sections of the thyroid show a lobulated parenchyma. Throughout the thyroid
parenchyma multiple small nodules composed of atypical aborted follicles are seen
lined by severe atypical epithelial cells. There is very scant colloid seen. The
larger nodule has a dense fibrous connective tissue with many satellite nodules
composed of similar atypical aborted follicles. There is evidence of vascular
invasion. Elsewhere the thyroid parenchyma shows severe chronic inflammatory cell
infiltration. Areas of hemorrhages are present. Other fragments contain mostly
lymphoid tissue with multiple nests of atypical aborted thyroid follicles.

Sections of the jugular vein show an intact wall.

SUMMARY:

THYROID TISSUE: FOLLICULAR CARCINOMA WITH EVIDENCE OF VASCULAR AND CAPSULAR
                  INVASION, MULTIPLE SATELLITE TUMOR NODULES ALL OVER THYROID TISSUE,
                  CHRONIC THYROIDITIS.
PORTION OF ANTERIOR JUGULAR VEIN: AN INTACT VEIN.
                          96-8333

Received: 8/20/86
Completed: 8/22/86 PC/nr
GH-109 REV. 10-81   P. Cruz, M.D./

About the Author

Nicholas James Gonzalez, MD, age 67, passed away suddenly at his home in New York City with his wife, Mary Beth, at his side. Born in Flushing, New York, he graduated from Brown University, Phi Beta Kappa, magna cum laude, with a degree in English Literature. He subsequently worked as a journalist, first at *Time*, Inc., before pursuing premedical studies at Columbia. He then received his medical degree from Cornell University Medical College in 1983. During a post-graduate immunology fellowship under Dr. Robert A. Good, considered the father of immunology, he completed a research study evaluating an aggressive nutritional therapy in the treatment of advanced cancer.

Dr. Gonzalez had been in private practice in New York City since 1987, treating patients diagnosed with cancer and other serious degenerative illnesses. His nutritional research has received substantial financial support from Proctor and Gamble and Nestle. Results from a pilot study published in 1999, described the most positive data in the medical literature for pancreatic cancer.

Dr. Gonzalez is the author of several books published by New Spring Press:
- *The Trophoblast and the Origins of Cancer*
- *One Man Alone: An Investigation of Nutrition, Cancer and Dr. William Donald Kelley*
- *The Enzyme Treatment of Cancer and Its Scientific Basis by Dr. John Beard, foreword by Dr. Gonzalez*
- *What Went Wrong: The Truth Behind The Clinical Trial of the Enzyme Treatment of Cancer.* **Independent Book Publishers Association 2013 Silver Award Winner**
- *Conquering Cancer: Volume One—50 Pancreatic and Breast Cancer Patients on The Gonzalez Nutritional Protocol*
- *Conquering Cancer: Volume Two—62 Patients on The Gonzalez Protocol*
- *Nutrition and The Autonomic Nervous System: The Scientific Foundations of The Gonzalez Protocol.* **2018 Book Excellence Award Winner for Diet and Nutrition**
- PLUS THE OFFICIAL NICHOLAS JAMES GONZALEZ, M.D. BIOGRAPHY TO BE RELEASED IN 2020

Dr. Nicholas Gonzalez leaves a legacy of faith, healing and genuine love for the truth, people and the pursuit of medicine. For more information about Dr. Gonzalez and The Gonzalez Protocol, visit The Nicholas Gonzalez Foundation website at www.thegonzalezprotocol.com

Books by Nicholas J. Gonzalez, M.D.
available on Amazon by New Spring Press

The Trophoblast and the Origins of Cancer

One Man Alone: An Investigation of Nutrition, Cancer and Dr. William Donald Kelley

The Enzyme Treatment of Cancer and Its Scientific Basis by
Dr. John Beard, foreword by Dr. Gonzalez

What Went Wrong: The Truth Behind The Clinical Trial of the Enzyme Treatment
of Cancer. Independent Book Publishers Association 2013 Silver Award Winner

Conquering Cancer: Volume One—50 Pancreatic and Breast
Cancer Patients on The Gonzalez Nutritional Protocol

Conquering Cancer: Volume Two—62 Patients on The Gonzalez Protocol

Nutrition and The Autonomic Nervous System: The Scientific Foundations of The
Gonzalez Protocol. 2018 Book Excellence Award Winner for Diet and Nutrition

Plus the official Nicholas James Gonzalez, M.D. biography to be released in 2020

Additional Patient Status: As of 2016

Dr. Nicholas Gonzalez also wrote a best-selling cancer case book series: ***Conquering Cancer Volume I and II***. This book was published in 2016 and represents the best cancer cases of Dr. Gonzalez's career—total of **112 patients on The Gonzalez Protocol with 17 different types of cancer**.

Thirteen of the same patients from ***Proof of Concept*** were included in the ***Conquering Cancer*** series. Since their patient status had been updated for that book in 2016, below is their updated patient status using the same patient coding as this book:

AF: Died August 1996 after quit program in April 1994 and stopped all treatment.

LJ: Survival 16+ years, and still alive.

LG: Survival 25.7+ years and still alive.

SH: Survived 6.5 years, died April 1998.

WC: Survived 22.1+ years and still alive.

LK: Last formal contact with Dr. Gonzalez was Feb 1997; however note in her file that states she is still alive and a 16+ year survivor.

DD: Died after surviving 18 years.

SA: Lost contact, 8+ month survivor of brain metastases from primary lung neoplasm.

MJ: A 24+ year survivor.

KG: A 21.2+ year survivor.

MW: A 16 year survivor who died in June 2004.

NR: A 25.6+ year survivor.

FA: A survivor of 12+ years who was lost to follow-up. Last contact in January 2002 and she claimed "excellent health".

The Nicholas Gonzalez Foundation

Founded in 2015, The Nicholas Gonzalez Foundation is keeping the brilliant, healing work of Nicholas J. Gonzalez, M.D. alive today and for generations to come. The foundation fuels the future of Dr. Gonzalez's legacy by preserving, promoting and propagating his holistic individualized nutrition protocols in the education about the treatment and prevention of cancer and other degenerative diseases.

We strive to inspire, guide and educate professional healers and patients on their path to discovering and adopting effective nutritional protocols for prevention and disease treatment.

Please consider supporting our mission with your prayers and financial assistance. There is a treasure trove of free information and videos about Dr. Gonzalez and The Gonzalez Protocol® at www.thegonzalezprotocol.com